in the mood for
QUICK FAMILY FOOD

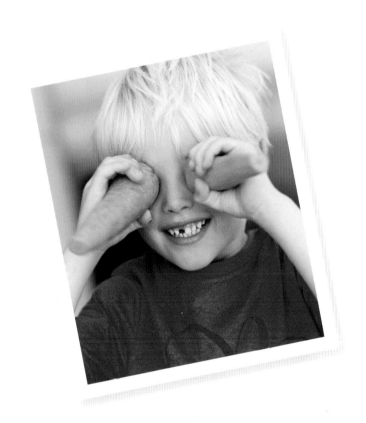

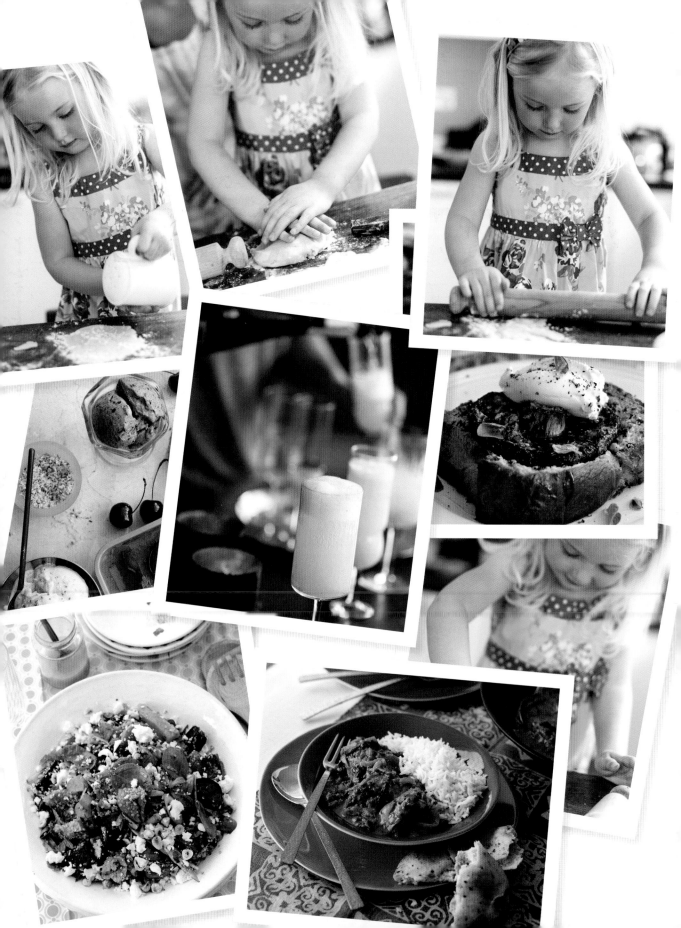

in the mood for
QUICK FAMILY FOOD

Simple, Fast and Delicious Recipes for Every Family

Jo Pratt

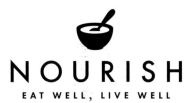

NOURISH

EAT WELL, LIVE WELL

IN THE MOOD FOR QUICK FAMILY FOOD
Jo Pratt

This edition published in the UK and USA in 2016
by Nourish, an imprint of Watkins Media Limited
19 Cecil Court
London WC2N 4EZ

enquiries@nourishbooks.com

First published in the United Kingdom and Ireland in 2013
as *Madhouse Cookbook* by Duncan Baird Publishers

Copyright © Watkins Media Limited 2013, 2016
Text and recipes copyright © Jo Pratt 2013, 2016
Photography copyright © Watkins Media Limited 2013, 2016

Managing Editor: Grace Cheetham
Editor: Wendy Hobson
Art Direction and Designer: Manisha Patel
Production: Uzma Taj
Commissioned Photography: Gareth Morgans
Food Stylist: Jo Pratt
Prop Stylist: Wei Tang

A CIP record for this book is available from the British Library

ISBN: 978-1-84899-294-8

10 9 8 7 6 5 4 3 2 1

Typeset in Myriad Pro
Colour reproduction by PDQ, UK
Printed in Bosnia & Herzegovina

DEDICATION
To madhouse proprietors everywhere

PUBLISHER'S NOTE
While every care has been taken in compiling the recipes for
this book, Watkins Media Limited, or any other persons
who have been involved in working on this publication, cannot
accept responsibility for any errors or omissions, inadvertent
or not, that may be found in the recipes or text, nor for any
problems that may arise as a result of preparing one of these
recipes. It is important that you consult a medical professional
before following any of the recipes or information contained
in this book if you have any special dietary requirements or
medical conditions. Ill or elderly people, babies, young children
and women who are pregnant or breastfeeding should avoid
recipes containing raw meat or uncooked eggs.

Notes on the recipes
Unless otherwise stated:
• Use large eggs
• Use medium fruit and vegetables
• Use fresh ingredients, including herbs and chillies
• Do not mix metric and imperial measurements
• 1 tsp = 5ml   1 tbsp = 15ml   1 cup = 250ml

ACKNOWLEDGEMENTS
A huge thanks to everyone who helped make this book…
    My children, Oliver and Rosa, and my husband Phil – the real
reasons the madhouse idea came about. The tears and tantrums
(mostly mine) have been worth it! All my family and friends for
your inspiration, ideas and taste buds.
    Everyone at Duncan Baird Publishers, in particular Grace
Cheetham, Wendy Hobson and Manisha Patel, for loving the
idea and making it great. Plus everyone in sales, marketing and
publicity for getting this book on bookshelves and in people's
homes. Gareth Morgans, Wei Tang, Poppy Campbell and Adrian
Lawrence for making everything on the photo shoot look so
fantastic and keeping it real.
    Thanks to Borra Garson and the team at DML for their
continued support in making things happen.
    Finally, a great big thanks to everyone who buys this book.
I hope it makes life less stressful in your madhouse.

PICTURE CREDIT
Wooden backgrounds pages 10–11, 76–77, 156–157:
Ingvar Bjork/Shutterstock

nourishbooks.com

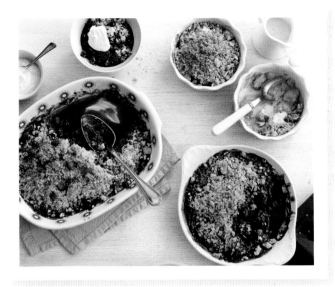

contents

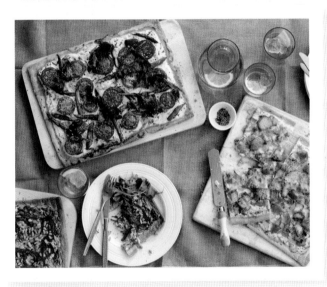

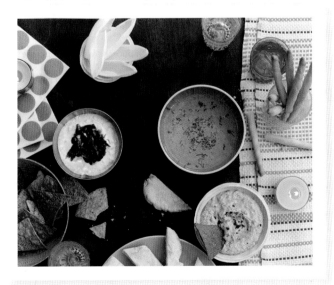

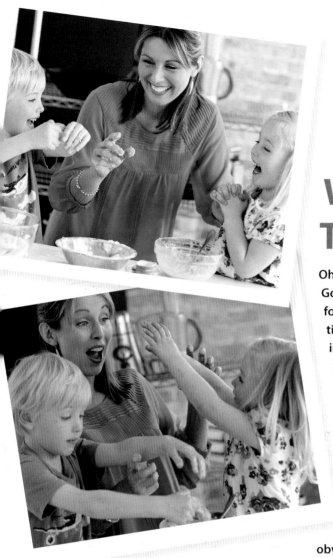

WELCOME TO
THE MADHOUSE

Oh, how my life has changed over the last few years. Gone are the days of spending a day or two preparing for elaborate dinner parties and cooking at random times when I felt like it and just because I could, with ingredients I hunted down in back-street markets and delicatessens.

That was all pre-children – now things are very different. I'm a busy mum who has to juggle work, children and all the associated chaos. I live in a madhouse! I'm always pushed for time, but I want to continue cooking food for me, my family and my friends, so it has to be simple, quick to prepare and easy to shop for – and I know I'm not alone here. Just reading around numerous websites and magazines, and chatting to other parents, it's obvious that most people find cooking for their families a challenge and just plain hard work.

I've taken a realistic look at the situations and circumstances that cooking for the whole family entails, and it certainly isn't as straightforward as just breakfast, lunch and dinner. There are times during the week, for example, when everyone is in such a rush getting to and from work/nursery/school/clubs that leave you feeling like a chef in a fast-food restaurant.

There are those occasions when you have no time to shop at the supermarket, so having a stack of meals in the freezer and ideas to cook from your storecupboard, or using ingredients you grab from your local shop or petrol station (if you are really desperate) are a necessity.

Other situations include those rare social get-togethers where you attempt to cling on to some sort of normality and have friends over for a good old gossipy (made easy) dinner party. And, of course, some great ideas for when you get a bit of quality time

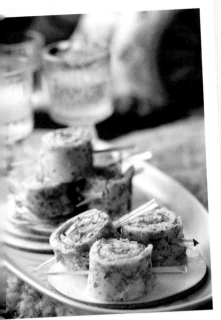

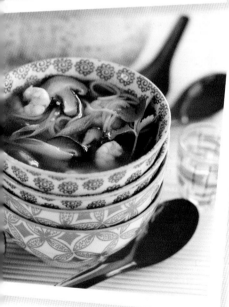

with your other half on a Saturday night and want something delicious to eat before you both fall asleep halfway through a film you've rented out.

So to reflect that new lifestyle, I have created three main chapters – Monday to Friday Survival, The Busy Weekend and Cling on to Your Social Life.

Monday to Friday Survival is, quite literally, recipes to help you get through the week of racing about and constantly chasing your tail. There are three sections to this chapter. Firstly, The Need for Speed, which is full of recipes that can be prepared and cooked very quickly. I'll often find that I have a 10-minute window to get my kids something to eat before they start rummaging through cupboards for snacks or have a meltdown due to hunger. But it's not just the kids who need food, fast. Once they're in bed, my husband and I also need to eat before it's too late (and we have a meltdown) so there are recipes that can be converted from a kids' meal to a grown-up meal. The second section is Quick Prep – Leave to Cook. Here you'll see one-pot dishes that require more lengthy cooking times so are perfect to make before school pick-up, or to prepare while the kids are eating their tea so the meal is ready for us to eat when they're in bed. Thirdly, Speedy Sweet Treats – so much more fun and interesting than the usual fruit or yogurt options, you'll find delicious choices like Lifesaver Speedy Chocolate Pudding and Fruity Fools with a Hidden Surprise.

So, you've survived the week, but as much as you look forward to the weekend, a family house is never a quiet house. Weekends seem to be at least as busy as the weeks and we tend to complicate them by upscaling everything and often trying to fit in more than there's room for. So The Busy Weekend covers some delicious Breakfasts to give your day a great start. Then there's a section of Light Bites so you can create easy lunchtime recipes, some of which use the bare minimum for when you've not had a chance to visit the supermarket or you've forgotten to book your online delivery, including tasty soups and snacks. These include imaginative meals from what you can find in the store cupboard.

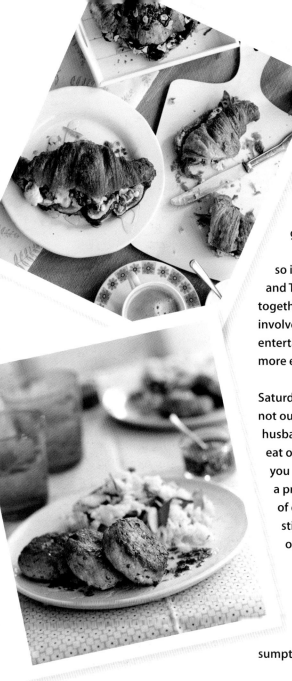

When you can all sit down together to share a meal, rather than eating in shifts as you tend to during the week, go to The Family Meal options for recipes you'll all enjoy.

Baking is a fun aspect to the weekend for my family so if you are like me, you might head straight for Baking and Things for a Sweet Tooth to find all kinds of cakes to bake together, including a couple of classic birthday cakes. Kids can get involved in many of the recipes in this chapter, which I find is good entertainment for them and a great way of getting them to be more experimental in the foods they eat.

Finally, a very important part of the weekend to me is Saturday Night – and the title says it all: Kids Are Banned. If we're not out (which is certainly less often now we have a family), my husband Phil and I will put more thought and effort into what we eat on a Saturday night so I've selected some delicious recipes you can cook together for starters and nibbles to enjoy with a pre-dinner drink, interesting main courses and a couple of desserts for a bit of delightful self-indulgence. These are all still quick and easy to prepare but with far less urgency than on week nights.

The final chapter, Cling on to Your Social Life, is packed with relaxed recipes for when you're doing some entertaining, many of which can be prepared ahead of time. There are some fabulous drinks and cocktails, nibbles and starters, impressive yet stress-free main courses and sumptuous desserts.

But let's be practical, you're not necessarily going to do a full-on dinner party every time you invite people over, so I've made sure you can tap in and out of these sections to suit the time you have available and the energy you have left! Something as simple as having friends over for a takeaway can be given a real lift if you start by welcoming them with a cocktail or offer home-made dips that took just a few minutes to prepare.

Time, however, is not always on your side, so look out for my Lifesavers – fabulous recipes that you can retrieve from your freezer or store cupboard to bring to the rescue when you are at a loss for what to serve. Dotted throughout the book, you'll find recipes like Savoury Crumbs, an amazingly versatile mixture to make up and

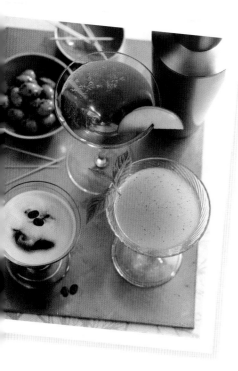

store in the freezer, plus things like my great cookie dough and freezer-to-pan salmon marinade.

Making your freezer and store cupboard your friend for life is one of the best things you can do to help you keep control in your madhouse. Having them well stocked will get you out of a hole on numerous occasions. So I've made sure there are plenty of recipes you can turn to that simply rely on a few basic ingredients from your store cupboard when you think the cupboard is bare! Plus I've added some simple How to Make recipes that are unbelievably easy and quick, but just as delicious as more complicated options.

You'll soon see that this book is all about being practical with your time, physical energy and the recipes and ingredients you choose. I hate wasting food so a really important part of these recipes is offering you recipes, tips and creative ideas on what to do with any Leftovers, whether it's making a lunchbox meal for the next day, creating a whole new meal for the freezer by adding a few additional ingredients, or even making a breakfast cereal out of your weekend baking once it's past its best – all of which make good use of time. You'll be amazed at just what you can make out of your leftovers and pop in the freezer for another day. Fill the rest of your freezer with plenty of frozen fruit and veg, ready-prepared pastry, bread, meat and fish.

My main piece of advice to avoid getting stressed out when cooking is to take a moment and read through the recipes before making them as – if your house is anything like mine – you're bound to be distracted by someone or something while you are actually cooking. If you don't have certain ingredients, don't panic. Try to be relaxed and practical about what ingredients you do have – be creative and substitute.

So, here's to being the ultimate mum and dad, the best hosts and *über* partners. Happy juggling and enjoy!

Jo Pratt
x

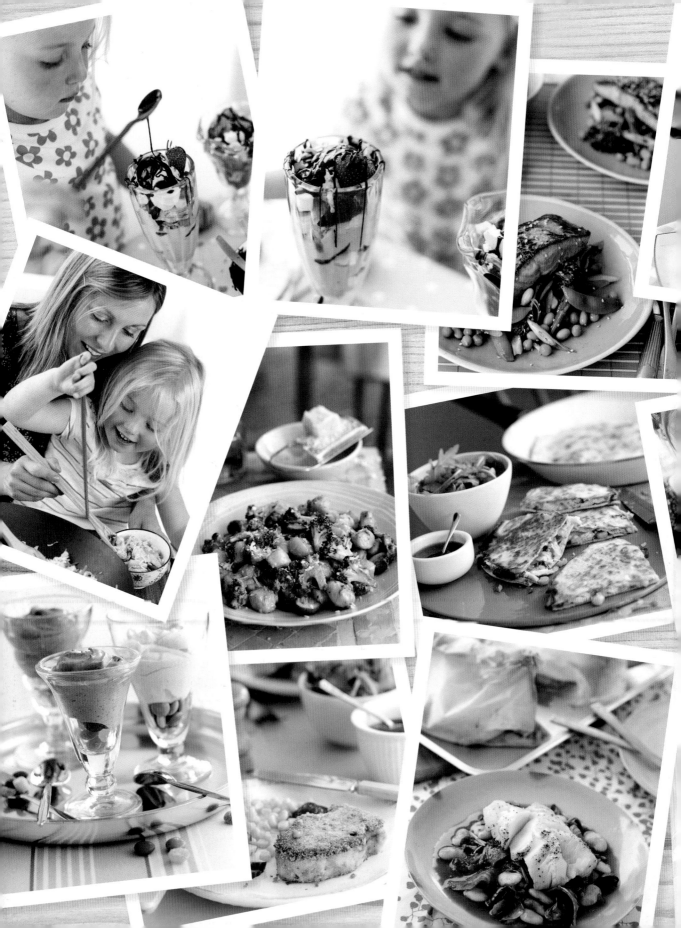

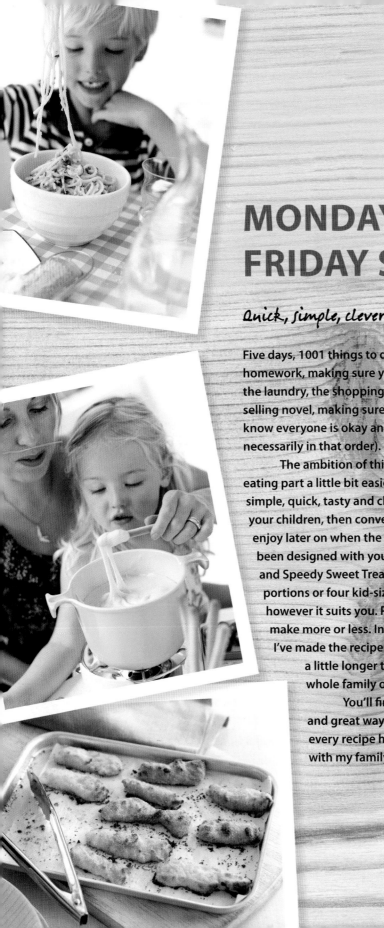

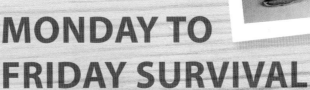

MONDAY TO FRIDAY SURVIVAL

Quick, simple, clever and delicious ...

Five days, 1001 things to do ... work, school, after-school clubs, homework, making sure you watch your favourite TV show, the laundry, the shopping, the cleaning, finishing that best-selling novel, making sure you've called your parents to let them know everyone is okay and, of course, cooking and eating (not necessarily in that order).

The ambition of this section is to make the cooking and eating part a little bit easier and more enjoyable. The recipes are simple, quick, tasty and clever, with tips like how to cook a dish for your children, then convert it into something the grown-ups will enjoy later on when the kids are in bed. Even the quantities have been designed with your lifestyle in mind. In The Need for Speed and Speedy Sweet Treats, most of the recipes are for two adult portions or four kid-sized portions, so you can mix and match however it suits you. Plus, of course, they are easy to adjust to make more or less. In the Quick Prep – Leave to Cook section, I've made the recipes to serve more portions as they take a little longer to cook, so you have plenty to feed the whole family or extras to freeze for another day.

You'll find lots of other top tips, lifesaving ideas and great ways to use leftovers, too. And, of course, every recipe has been stress tested in my own kitchen with my family and they work ... no, they rock!

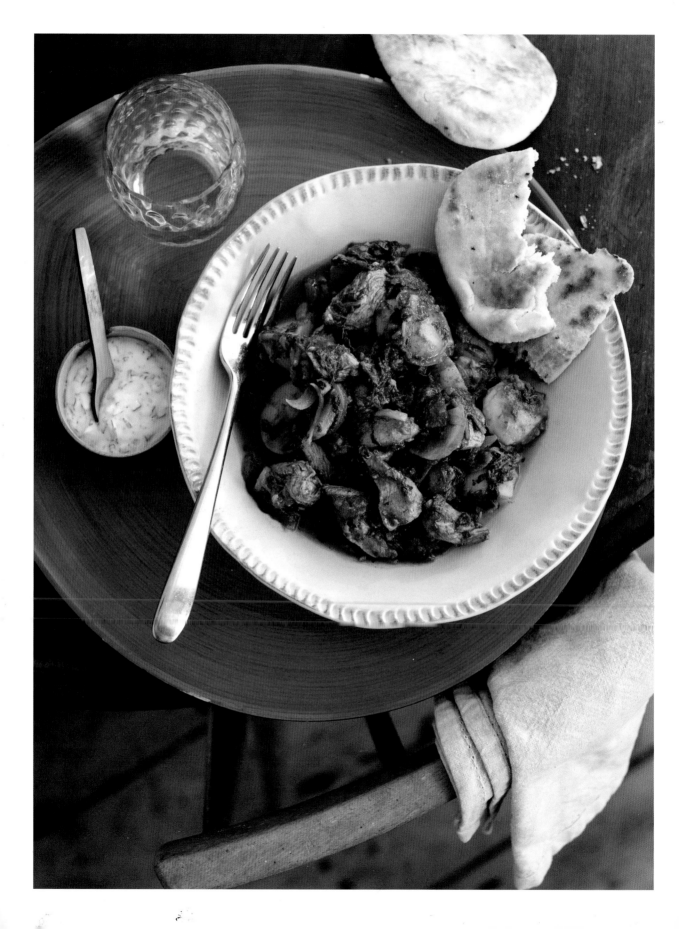

I love to make this recipe on a Friday night. It's great for using up leftover potatoes and can be made quicker than it takes to organize a take-out. I always keep a bag of frozen spinach in the freezer – it's really convenient for all sorts of dishes. If I have some fresh spinach in the refrigerator, though, I just roughly chop a couple of big handfuls and add them when the curry is almost ready.

Chicken, Potato and Spinach Curry in a Hurry

MAKES 2 adult or 4 kid-sized portions
PREPARATION TIME 10 minutes
COOKING TIME 20 minutes

1½ tbsp sunflower or vegetable oil
1 onion, thinly sliced
2 skinless chicken breasts, diced
2 garlic cloves, crushed
3–4cm/1¼–1½in piece of root ginger, peeled and grated
1 tbsp garam masala
½ tsp chilli powder
400g/14oz/1¾ cups canned chopped tomatoes
200g/7oz cooked new or salad potatoes, halved if large (canned potatoes are also fine)
150g/5½oz/1 cup frozen spinach, defrosted
sea salt and freshly ground black pepper

TO SERVE
naan bread
home-made Cucumber Raita (see page 25) or shop-bought raita
mango chutney

1 Heat the oil in a large pan over a low heat, add the onion and cook for a few minutes until soft. Increase the heat to medium, add the chicken, garlic and ginger and fry for 3–4 minutes until the chicken turns opaque. Stir in the garam masala and chilli powder and continue to cook for about 1 minute.

2 Add the tomatoes, potatoes and 150ml/5fl oz/scant ⅔ cup water. Bring to the boil, then reduce the heat, cover loosely with a lid and leave to simmer gently for about 10 minutes until the chicken is cooked through.

3 Stir in the spinach, season lightly with salt and pepper, then cook for a further 2–3 minutes, stirring occasionally.

4 Serve the curry on its own or with naan bread, raita and mango chutney, if you like.

Leftovers for the freezer
frozen ginger
If you have a large piece of **root ginger** left over, don't leave it lurking in the corner of your refrigerator to deteriorate gradually. Put all or some of it in a sandwich bag, seal, label and store in the freezer – it will keep for several months. When a recipe calls for grated ginger, it will grate really easily straight from frozen – no need to defrost or peel.

This is one of my kids' favourites and a great way to use up leftover rice. You can use ham or other favourites instead of the chicken, if you prefer, so you can be sure they'll love it.

Very Special Fried Rice

MAKES 2 adult or 4 kid-sized portions
PREPARATION TIME 10 minutes
COOKING TIME 7 minutes

2 skinless chicken breasts, thinly sliced
2 tbsp soy sauce
2 tbsp clear honey
1 tbsp sunflower or vegetable oil
4 spring onions/scallions, finely chopped
150g/5½oz green beans, cut into pieces
1 carrot or courgette/zucchini, peeled
  and coarsely grated
250g/9oz/1⅔ cups cooked basmati rice
  (either shop-bought pre-cooked or
  using leftovers)
75g/2½oz/scant ½ cup sweetcorn
100g/3½oz canned diced pineapple,
  drained
1 egg, beaten

1 Put the chicken breasts in a bowl and stir in the soy sauce and honey. Leave to one side to marinate for a few minutes.

2 Heat the oil in a wok over a medium heat, add the chopped and grated vegetables and stir-fry for about 1 minute. Add the chicken and the marinade and stir-fry for a few minutes until the chicken is cooked through. Add the rice, sweetcorn and pineapple and stir-fry for about 2 minutes until the rice is hot right through.

3 Pour in the egg, stirring to mix the egg through the rice, and fry for about 30 seconds.

4 Serve with chopsticks for an authentic touch (and the entertainment value in most cases).

How to cook
perfect basmati rice
Start with a good-quality basmati rice and measure out the amount you need. As a general rule, **1 part rice** to **2 parts water** is the ratio, so to make life easy, measure the quantity of rice in a cup and use the same one to measure the water. Unless a recipe states otherwise, **65g/2¼oz/⅓ cup is usually sufficient per adult portion**. Pop the rice in a sieve/fine-mesh strainer and rinse under the cold tap for about 1 minute to remove excess starch. Shake off as much water as you can, then tip the rice into a pan. Now measure in twice as much cold water and **a pinch of salt**. Bring to the boil over a high heat. Immediately reduce the heat to low, cover with a tight-fitting lid and leave untouched for 10 minutes. Turn off the heat and, with the lid still on, leave for a further 5 minutes. Run a fork through the rice and you will have delicious, fluffy basmati rice.

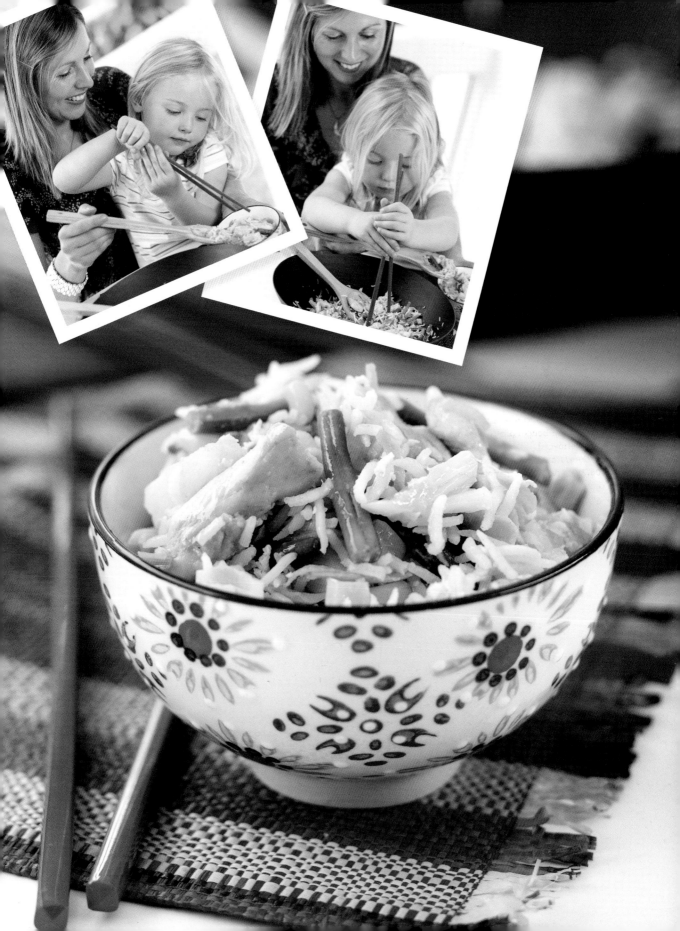

It's great to experiment with different filling options depending on what you like and can get your hands on. Just don't fill too much otherwise the quesadillas will be too difficult to flip over. It'll still taste good but it might look a bit battered! Our household favourite fillings include baked beans, grated Cheddar and a shake of Worcestershire sauce, or grated Cheddar with sliced avocado, fresh coriander/cilantro and tomato salsa.

Chicken, Cheese and Corn Quesa-d-easies

MAKES 2 adult or 4 kid-sized portions
PREPARATION TIME 5 minutes
COOKING TIME 12 minutes

4 flour or corn tortillas
1 handful of rocket/arugula leaves,
   to serve

**FOR THE CHICKEN, CHEESE AND CORN
   FILLING**
2 large handfuls of grated Cheddar
   cheese
2 large handfuls of leftover cooked
   chicken, torn into small pieces
4 tbsp sweetcorn
2 tbsp sweet chilli dipping sauce, plus
   extra for serving (optional)
1 tbsp chopped parsley leaves

1 Heat a frying pan to a medium heat. Put one tortilla in the pan and sprinkle over half of the filling ingredients. Cover with the second tortilla and cook for 2–3 minutes.

2 Gently turn the whole quesadilla over and cook for a further 2–3 minutes until the base is golden and the cheese has melted.

3 Remove the quesadilla from the pan and keep it warm while you cook the second one. Transfer them to a board and cut into quarters, using a pizza wheel if you have one. Serve hot with the rocket/arugula leaves and extra chilli dipping sauce, if you like.

Leftovers for a pizza
tortilla pizzas

This is the quickest, easiest pizza that kids (and grown-ups) of all ages will enjoy. Simply spread **1 tbsp tomato purée/paste** or **sun-dried tomato purée/paste** onto a piece of **tortilla bread**. Scatter over some **grated Cheddar cheese** (or half Cheddar and half grated mozzarella). Leave plain or add **chopped ham**, **salami**, **shredded chicken**, **drained and flaked canned tuna**, **sliced olives**, **sweetcorn**, **sliced onion** or **halved cherry tomatoes**. Don't add too much or the pizza will be top heavy. Put on a baking sheet and cook in a preheated oven at 220°C/425°F/gas 7 for 8–10 minutes until melted and just how you like it.

P.S. It is well worth making one more than you think you'll need of these as they will be gone in seconds!

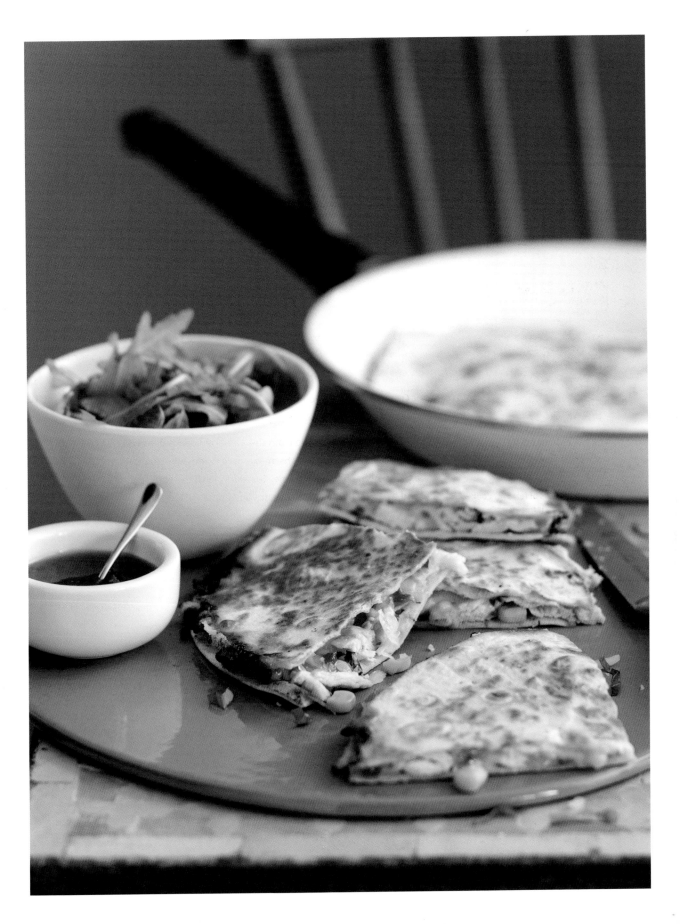

Here's one for all you lovers of yeast extract out there. Serve it with your favourite vegetables or, to make it a bit more grown up, in a chunk of ciabatta with rocket/arugula, guacamole (see below), sliced tomato and mayonnaise to make a sort of club sandwich.

Crunchy Love-it-or-Hate-it Chicken

MAKES 2 adult or 4 kid-sized portions
PREPARATION TIME 15 minutes using
   pre-made Savoury Crumbs or 25 minutes
   from scratch
COOKING TIME 5 minutes

2 skinless chicken breasts
1 egg white
2 tsp yeast extract
100g/3½oz/1 cup Savoury Crumbs
   (see page 30) or plain breadcrumbs
sunflower oil, for frying

TO SERVE
baked beans or vegetables of your
   choice
home-made Oven-baked Chips (see
   page 148) or shop-bought chips/fries,
   mashed potatoes or rice

1 Put the chicken breasts in between two sheets of baking paper and bash with a rolling pin to flatten slightly. Cut into 1–2cm/½–¾in strips.

2 Lightly beat the egg white and yeast extract together until just frothy. Add the chicken and leave for a couple of minutes.

3 Toss the chicken pieces, a few at a time, in the savoury crumbs. (Pieces of crumb-coated chicken can be frozen for up to 3 months. Defrost them thoroughly before frying.)

4 Meanwhile, pour enough oil into a frying pan to cover the surface and heat over a medium heat. Add the chicken pieces and fry for a couple of minutes on each side until golden, crunchy and cooked through. Drain on paper towels.

5 Serve with baked beans or vegetables and your favourite chips/fries, mashed potatoes or rice.

How to make

home-made guacamole

Put the flesh of **2 ripe avocados** in the bowl of a small food processor or suitable container for a hand blender. Remove the seeds from **1 tomato** and roughly chop the flesh, then add it to the avocados with **1 garlic clove**, the **juice of ½ lime** and **a few coriander/cilantro leaves**. Whizz to a rough or smooth consistency. If you want some spice, add **1 deseeded and finely chopped red chilli** or **a few good splashes of Tabasco sauce**. For some crunch, add **½ finely chopped red onion**. Season to taste with **sea salt** and **freshly ground black pepper** before serving. If you are not planning to serve the guacamole straight away, put the avocado stone into the finished guacamole to help prevent it from going brown. Covered with cling film/plastic wrap, it will store in the refrigerator for a day.

We all resort to pasta recipes for quick and easy meals – so here's another to add to your repertoire. It's one of those dishes that I'll cook when we're in the mood for comfort food, and the ingredients are usually sitting in my refrigerator. If I don't have any cream, then crème fraîche or plain yogurt make a convenient substitute.

Bacon, Leek and Brie Penne

MAKES 2 adult or 4 kid-sized portions
PREPARATION TIME 10 minutes
COOKING TIME 15 minutes

250g/9oz/2¾ cups penne
a drizzle of olive oil
100g/3½oz bacon lardons or pancetta, diced
1 leek, sliced
100ml/3½fl oz/scant ½ cup white wine
100ml/3½fl oz/scant ½ cup single/light cream
100g/3½oz Brie, cut into small chunks
a pinch of dried chilli/hot pepper flakes
sea salt and plenty of freshly ground black pepper

1 Bring a large pan of lightly salted water to the boil, add the penne and return to the boil. Leave to simmer for about 10 minutes until just tender.

2 Meanwhile, heat the oil in a large frying pan over a medium heat, add the bacon and fry for 5 minutes until golden. Drain off any excess fat, then add the leek to the pan. Fry over a low heat for 5 minutes until softened. Pour in the wine and bring to the boil. Stir in the cream, Brie, chilli/hot pepper flakes and black pepper.

3 Drain the pasta and add to the sauce. Stir gently over a low heat for about a minute or so, then serve.

Leftover lardons
spicy bacon and tomato sauce
If you had to open a large pack of lardons or pancetta, it's well worth making a quick pasta sauce for the refrigerator or freezer. Fry the **lardons** in a **drizzle of olive oil** until golden. Add a **can of chopped tomatoes** and **a good pinch each of dried chilli/hot pepper flakes** and **dried oregano**. Simmer for 10 minutes until thickened. Stir in **2 tbsp mascarpone** or **cream cheese** and some **sea salt** and **freshly ground black pepper**, then keep in the refrigerator for a couple of days or in the freezer for up to 3 months. Heat up and toss with cooked pasta.

We love carbonara in our house, but the rich, creamy version is sometimes a bit too much for midweek. Try this lighter option if you're a fan – it even contributes to one of your five a day.

Spaghetti and Courgette Carbonara

MAKES 2 adult or 4 kid-sized portions
PREPARATION TIME 15 minutes
COOKING TIME 12 minutes

250g/9oz spaghetti
1 tbsp olive oil
125g/4½oz/scant 1 cup finely diced smoked streaky bacon
1 courgette/zucchini, grated
1 garlic clove, crushed
2 eggs, lightly beaten
100g/3½oz mascarpone
25g/1oz/¼ cup freshly grated Parmesan cheese
sea salt and freshly ground black pepper

1 Bring a large pan of lightly salted water to the boil, add the spaghetti and return to the boil. Leave to simmer for about 10 minutes until it is just tender.

2 Meanwhile, heat the oil in a large frying pan over a medium heat, add the bacon and fry for 5–8 minutes until golden. Add the courgette/zucchini and garlic and fry for a couple of minutes to take away the initial rawness.

3 In a bowl, mix together the eggs, mascarpone and Parmesan and season lightly with salt and pepper.

4 As soon as the spaghetti is cooked, remove it from the water with a pair of tongs and put it straight into the pan with the bacon and courgette/zucchini and toss around. Finally, add the egg mixture.

5 Remove from the heat and toss together to coat the spaghetti in the sauce. The heat from the spaghetti will cook the egg just enough without it scrambling. Serve immediately.

Leftovers transformed
spaghetti fritters

Any leftover spaghetti carbonara can be transformed into really tasty fritters that are perfect for lunch or even cold in school lunchboxes. Simply take the leftovers and snip the **spaghetti** a couple of times with a pair of scissors into smaller pieces. Mix with enough **beaten egg** to bind. You can also add some **peas**, **sweetcorn** or more **grated courgette/zucchini** here too. Heat **a drizzle of olive oil** in a frying pan. Add spoonfuls of the spaghetti mixture and fry until golden on both sides. Drain on paper towels and serve hot or cold.

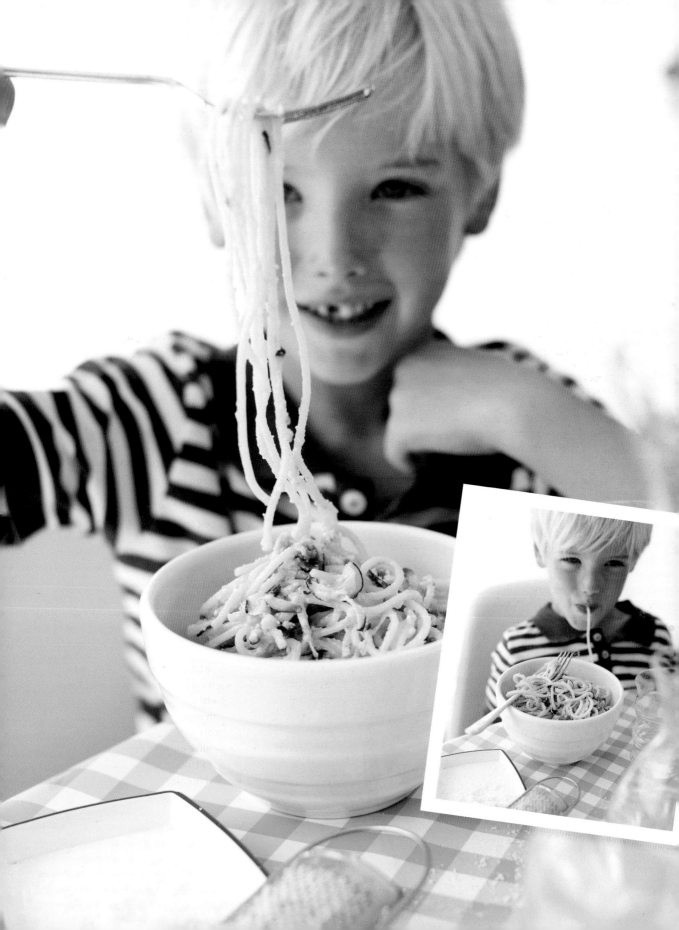

This is great recipe that can be cooked up as a family meal or, once you have prepared everything, you can halve the mixture and cook one half for the kids to enjoy as a teatime treat and the other for a grown-up meal a bit later on. It's ideal for using up leftover potatoes, and it really doesn't matter if they break up when you chop them. They will go even crunchier that way.

Corned Beef and Sweetcorn Hash with a Dash of Flexibility

MAKES 2 adult or 4 kid-sized portions
PREPARATION TIME 10 minutes
COOKING TIME 20 minutes

2–3 tbsp olive oil
1 onion, finely sliced
400g/14oz cooked potatoes, cut into small chunks
340g/11¾oz canned corned beef, crumbled into chunks
200g/7oz canned sweetcorn, drained
a shake of Worcestershire sauce
a pinch of dried chilli/hot pepper flakes (optional)
2 handfuls of baby spinach leaves, roughly chopped (or use frozen)
sea salt and freshly ground black pepper

TO SERVE
fried or poached eggs (optional)
sweet chilli sauce, tomato ketchup or brown sauce

1 Heat 1 tbsp of the oil in a frying pan, add the onion and fry over a low heat for about 5 minutes until it softens and starts to turn golden.

2 Transfer to a bowl and add the potatoes, corned beef, sweetcorn, Worcestershire sauce and chilli/hot pepper flakes, if using. Season lightly with salt and pepper. Mix to combine and either divide into individual portions or cook as one large hash. (The hash can be divided into portions before cooking and any that isn't cooked straight away can be kept in the refrigerator for later.)

3 Heat the remaining oil in the frying pan over a medium-high heat, add the hash and cook for about 5 minutes, stirring to heat everything through. Stir the spinach into the mixture and continue to fry for about 5 minutes, stirring just until everything is hot, then without stirring for about 5 minutes or so, until the corned beef and potatoes turn golden brown and crisp up at the edges.

4 Serve as it is or topped with a fried or poached egg, if you like, and a sauce of your choice.

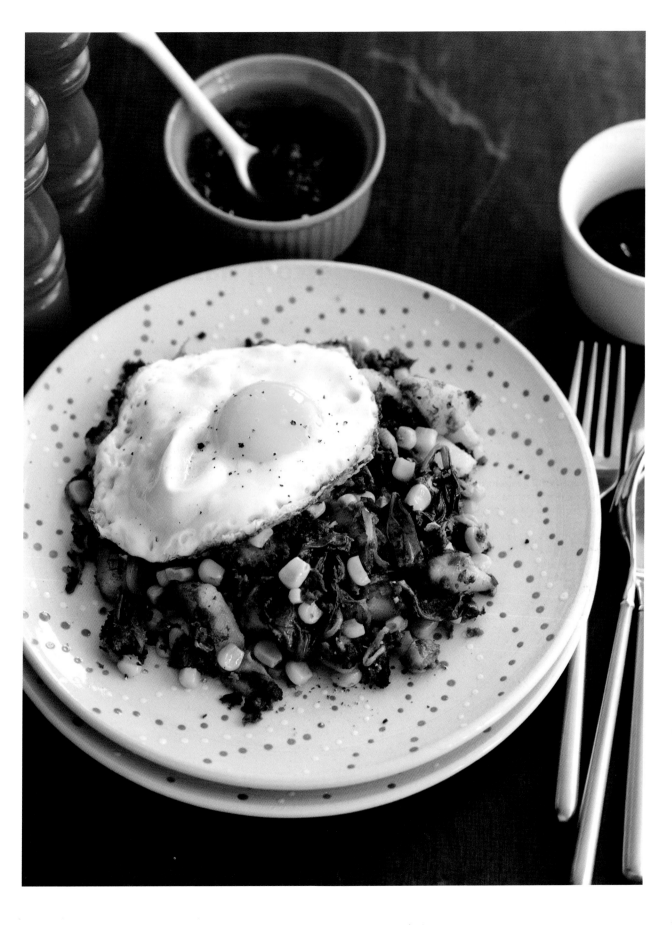

Serve this super-speedy steak sarnie and you'll be in everyone's good books. The crucial ingredient is the pan-fried avocado – oddly, it smells and tastes like bacon! Chips/fries are a great accompaniment – you can make your own (see page 148) or just throw in some shop-bought chips/fries – I find the thinner variety cook better in the oven as they go crunchier than the fatter versions. Oh and use any bread you have to hand – you don't have to use posh bread.

Speedy Steak and Pan-fried Avocado Club Sarnie

MAKES 2 adult or 4 kid-sized portions
PREPARATION TIME 10 minutes
COOKING TIME 5 minutes

1 tbsp Dijon mustard
1 tbsp clear honey
a shake of Worcestershire sauce
2 minute steaks
a drizzle of olive oil
1 small avocado, pitted, peeled and
   sliced
6 slices of bread
¼ small iceberg lettuce, shredded
2 tbsp mayonnaise
a squeeze of lemon juice
2 tomatoes, thinly sliced
sea salt and freshly ground black pepper

TO SERVE
home-made Oven-baked Chips (see
   page 148) or shop-bought chips/fries
home-made Perfect Coleslaw (see page
   93) or shop-bought coleslaw

1 Mix together the mustard, honey and Worcestershire sauce, then spread or brush the mixture over both sides of the steaks.

2 Heat a griddle or frying pan over a high heat until hot enough to start to smoke. Put the steaks in the hot pan and cook for about 1 minute on each side (depending on their thickness) until golden. At the same time, drizzle the oil over the sliced avocado and season lightly with salt and pepper. Fry in the same pan for 1–2 minutes on each side until golden.

3 Meanwhile, lightly toast the bread on both sides.

4 Mix the lettuce with the mayonnaise and lemon juice and divide half the mixture between two pieces of the toast. Top them with the pan-fried avocado and then with a second piece of toast. Spread the remaining lettuce on top, then add the steak. Add the tomatoes, season lightly with salt and pepper, then finish with the last pieces of toast. Press down lightly.

5 Cut in half or into quarters, secure with cocktail sticks/toothpicks and serve with chips/fries and coleslaw.

I find that Monday to Friday survival is a little easier when I'm cooking with one pan. There are fewer distractions and therefore fewer things that can go wrong. Just follow the step-by-step methods and the results will be delicious. If you don't have smoked salmon, try this with smoked mackerel or trout. You can even use pieces of leftover roast chicken, turkey or lamb, which are equally delicious. It is also a good way to use up leftover rice.

One-pan Hot-smoked Salmon Biryani

MAKES 2 adult or 4 kid-sized portions
PREPARATION TIME 15 minutes
COOKING TIME 15 minutes

1 tbsp sunflower oil
1 onion, finely sliced
2 garlic cloves, crushed
2cm/¾in piece of root ginger, peeled and grated
1 handful of sultanas/golden raisins
1 tbsp garam masala
200g/7oz broccoli, tenderstem, asparagus, green beans or mangetout/snow peas cut into chunks
250g/9oz/1²⁄₃ cups cooked brown or white basmati rice
150g/5½oz hot-smoked salmon fillets, flaked into pieces
1 handful of toasted flaked/slivered almonds
a squeeze of lemon juice
4 tbsp plain yogurt, crème fraîche or sour cream
1 small handful of coriander/cilantro, dill or mint leaves, chopped
sea salt and freshly ground black pepper

1 Heat the oil in a large frying pan over a low heat and fry the onion for about 5 minutes until becoming golden. Stir in the garlic, ginger, sultanas/golden raisins and garam masala and cook for a further 1 minute. Add the green vegetables and fry together for about 2–3 minutes until the vegetables are just tender.

2 Stir in the rice, salmon and almonds. Season lightly with salt and pepper. Stir-fry over a medium heat for a few minutes until the rice and salmon are heated through.

3 Gently stir through the lemon juice, yogurt and herbs and serve immediately.

How to make

cucumber raita

Blend together **150ml/5fl oz/scant ²⁄₃ cup Greek yogurt**, **¼ cucumber**, seeds removed, **1 small handful of chopped mint** or **coriander/cilantro leaves** and **a pinch of sea salt** until well combined. Serve straight away or you can keep it in the refrigerator for up to a day.

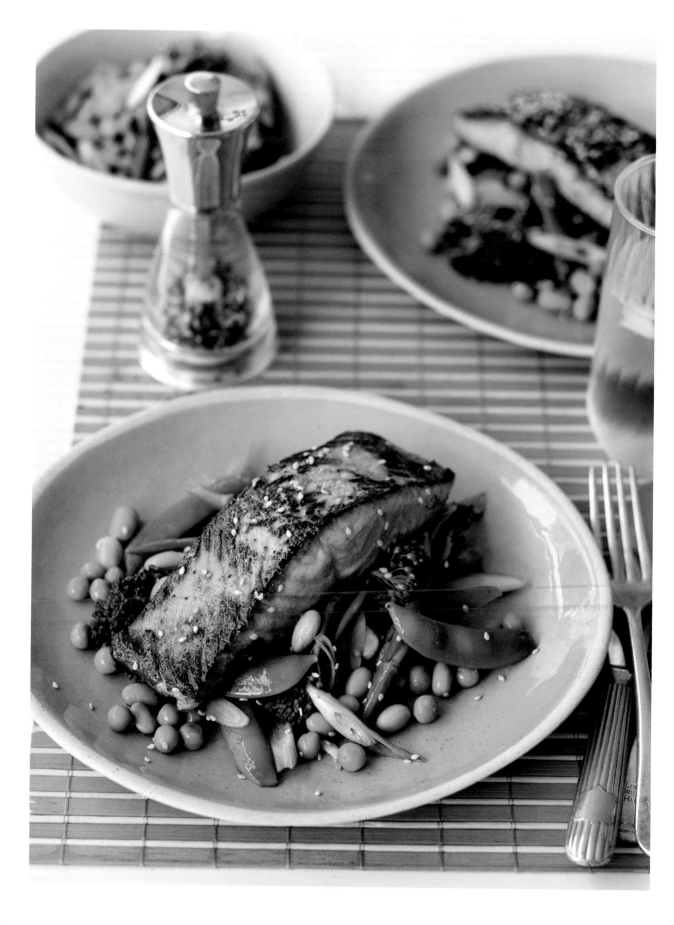

Marinate the salmon while you're getting the kids' school bags ready for the next day, polishing school shoes, washing sports kit (and hoping it will dry in time) and making sure your kids have cleaned their teeth before they go to bed. Once that's all done, this is a delicious recipe for two that takes no time at all to whip up.

Honey Miso Salmon with Warm Green Salad

MAKES 2 adult or 4 kid-sized portions
PREPARATION TIME 10 minutes, plus at least 30 minutes marinating (optional)
COOKING TIME 5 minutes

FOR THE HONEY MISO SALMON
2 salmon fillets, skinned
½ recipe quantity Honey Miso Marinade (see below)
sunflower or olive oil, for brushing
1 tsp toasted sesame seeds

FOR THE WARM GREEN SALAD
200g/7oz broccoli or tenderstem broccoli
100g/3½oz sugar snap peas
85g/3oz/scant ½ cup frozen soy beans or broad beans, defrosted
85g/3oz/scant ⅔ cup frozen peas, defrosted
2 spring onions/scallions, finely sliced on an angle
juice of ½ lime
1 tsp toasted sesame oil
1 tbsp olive oil
1 small handful of coriander/cilantro leaves, chopped
sea salt and freshly ground black pepper

1 Put the salmon in a shallow, non-metallic bowl, pour over the marinade and rub it into the fillets. Cover and leave to marinate in the refrigerator for about 30 minutes, or longer if you can, but it can be cooked straight away if necessary.

2 Brush a frying pan or griddle with a little oil over a medium-high heat, add the salmon and cook for a couple of minutes on each side until just cooked through.

3 Meanwhile, bring a pan of water to the boil, put the broccoli and sugar snap peas in a steamer basket and steam for up to 5 minutes until tender.

4 Transfer to a bowl and toss with the remaining salad ingredients, seasoning lightly with salt and pepper.

5 Scatter the sesame seeds over the hot salmon and serve with the warm salad.

Lifesaver marinade
honey miso marinade
Make up a batch of this marinade and store in a jar in the refrigerator for up to 2 weeks. Use it to flavour fish, chicken, pork or beef before frying or grilling/broiling. These measurements will give you 4 adult portions, but you can prepare as much as you like. Mix together: **2 tbsp clear honey**, **2 tbsp miso paste**, **2 tsp rice vinegar** or **lime juice**, **2 tbsp light soy sauce** and **4cm/1½in piece of root ginger**, peeled and finely grated.

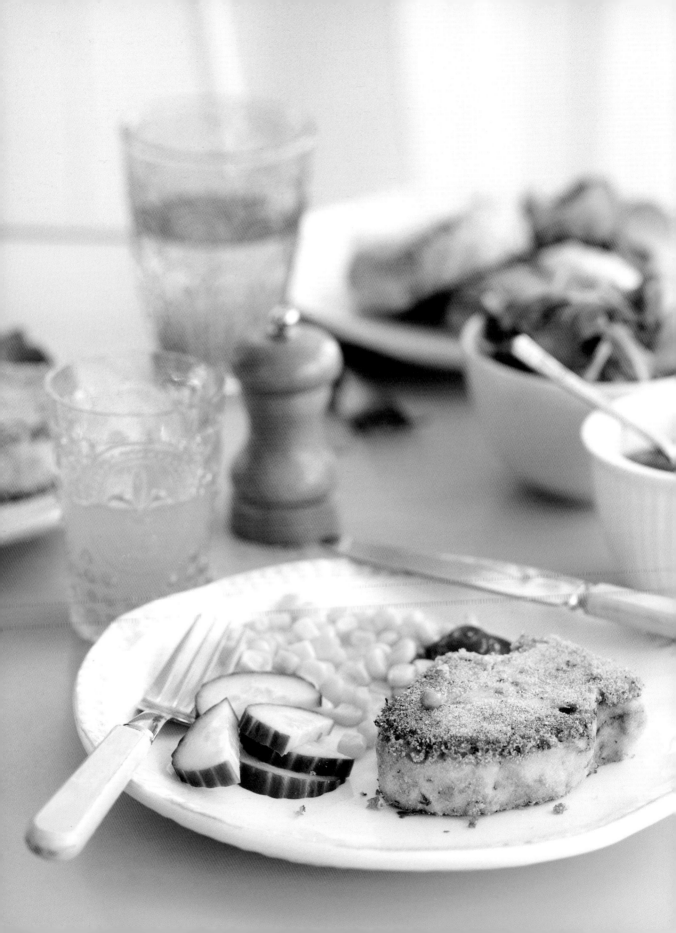

I've tried to write the recipes in this section using ingredients that most of us will have in our cupboards or refrigerators. There may be a few things you need to pick up at the supermarket but nothing out of the ordinary. For example, this recipe uses canned tuna, potatoes, frozen peas, olive oil, spring onions/scallions and lemons – all fairly standard staples – so all you need to remember to add to your shopping list is parsley (buy a growing pot) and some semolina or polenta (which will last ages), then these little beauties can be made as a lovely, quick midweek meal. Instead of tuna, try canned salmon or even leftover cooked salmon, cod or other white fish. Peas can be swapped for sweetcorn or mixed frozen veg, and other herbs can be used instead of parsley, such as chives, dill or tarragon.

Pea and Tuna Fishcakes with Caper and Lemon Mayonnaise

MAKES 2 adult or 4 kid-sized portions
PREPARATION TIME 15 minutes if using
   previously cooked mashed potato
COOKING TIME 10 minutes

300g/10½oz cooked potatoes
165g/5¾oz canned tuna, drained and
   flaked
4 spring onions/scallions, finely chopped
75g/2½oz/scant ½ cup frozen peas,
   defrosted
1 tbsp chopped parsley leaves
finely grated zest of 1 lemon
125g/4½oz/1 cup semolina or polenta
   (or 125g/4½oz/1¼ cups Savoury
   Crumbs on page 30)
3 tbsp olive oil
sea salt and freshly ground black pepper

FOR THE CAPER AND LEMON
   MAYONNAISE
4 tbsp mayonnaise
1 tbsp chopped capers
1 tbsp chopped parsley leaves
1 tbsp lemon juice
a pinch of cayenne pepper

TO SERVE
tomato ketchup or mayonnaise
mixed green salad

1 Put the potatoes in a large bowl and mash them. Add the tuna, spring onions/scallions, peas, parsley and lemon zest, and season lightly with salt and pepper. Mix until well combined.

2 Using wet hands to stop the mixture sticking to you, shape into fish cakes – large or small, it's up to you. Lightly coat each one all over with the semolina. (Cook straight away or chill until needed.)

3 Heat the oil in large frying pan over a medium heat, add the fishcakes and fry for 4–5 minutes on each side until golden. You may need to do this in a couple of batches, depending on the size of your frying pan. Take care not to have the heat too high as you want to make sure they are heated all the way through.

4 To make the mayonnaise, simply mix together all the ingredients. (Any leftovers will keep in the refrigerator for up to a week in a screw-topped jar.)

5 Serve the fishcakes with the caper mayonnaise (or kids will probably opt for ketchup or plain mayonnaise). They are great on their own or with a fresh salad.

This is what I call a flexi-recipe – either a family meal, or one where the kids eat earlier and the adults enjoy the meal (perhaps with a glass of wine) when the kids are in bed. Prepare and freeze the fish fingers ahead of time, then just cook when you need them.

Fish Finger Tortillas

MAKES 2 adult or 4 kid-sized portions
PREPARATION TIME 10 minutes using pre-made Savoury Crumbs or 20 minutes from scratch
COOKING TIME 6 minutes

FOR THE FISH FINGERS
250g/9oz thick fish fillet, such as salmon, cod, haddock, pollack or other white fish
2 tbsp plain/all-purpose flour
1 egg, lightly beaten
75g/2½oz/¾ cup Savoury Crumbs (see below)
2–3 tbsp olive oil
a pinch of sea salt (optional)

TO SERVE
tortilla bread or wraps
choose any accompaniment, including:
• shredded lettuce or rocket/arugula
• tomato salsa, hot pepper sauce, ketchup
• mayonnaise (flavoured with garlic, lime or lemon juice), sour cream
• sliced tomatoes
• sliced avocado
• Home-made Guacamole (see page 18) or shop-bought guacamole

1 Cut the fish into 12 finger shapes and season lightly with salt, if you like.

2 Put the flour, egg and savoury crumbs into three separate medium-sized sandwich bags or shallow bowls. First, coat the fish fingers, a few at a time, in flour, then egg and finally turn gently in the crumbs so they are evenly coated. (The fish fingers can be prepared to this stage and kept in the refrigerator for a day or frozen for up to 3 months.)

3 To cook, heat a frying pan over a medium heat and add the oil. If you plan on cooking just a few, use less oil. Once hot, add the fish fingers and cook for 2–3 minutes on each side until golden and cooked through. Alternatively, if you have the oven on (for example, to cook some chips/fries or potato wedges, see page 148), lightly toss the fish fingers in the oil, put on a hot baking sheet and cook for about 6 minutes until golden, turning halfway. (If cooking from frozen, add a couple of minutes on each side, and fry or bake until completely cooked through.)

4 Once the fish fingers are cooked, either warm your tortillas in the microwave or lightly toast under the grill/broiler, then tailor-make your tortillas to everyone's liking. Serve hot

Lifesaver for the freezer
savoury crumbs
Simply whizz **200g/7oz white bread** (with or without the crust) to a fine crumb in a food processor. Add **50g/1¾oz/⅓ cup polenta** or **semolina** and **50g/1¾oz/⅔ cup finely grated Parmesan cheese** and put into one large or a few smaller freezer bags. You can also shake in other flavourings before you freeze or add just before using, such as **grated lemon**, **lime** or **orange zest**, **chopped herbs**, **finely chopped nuts**, **dried herbs**, **garam masala**, **paprika**, **chilli powder**, **Chinese five-spice**, **jerk** or **Cajun seasoning**. When just frozen, shake the bag to break up the crumbs so they don't stay frozen in a solid clump.

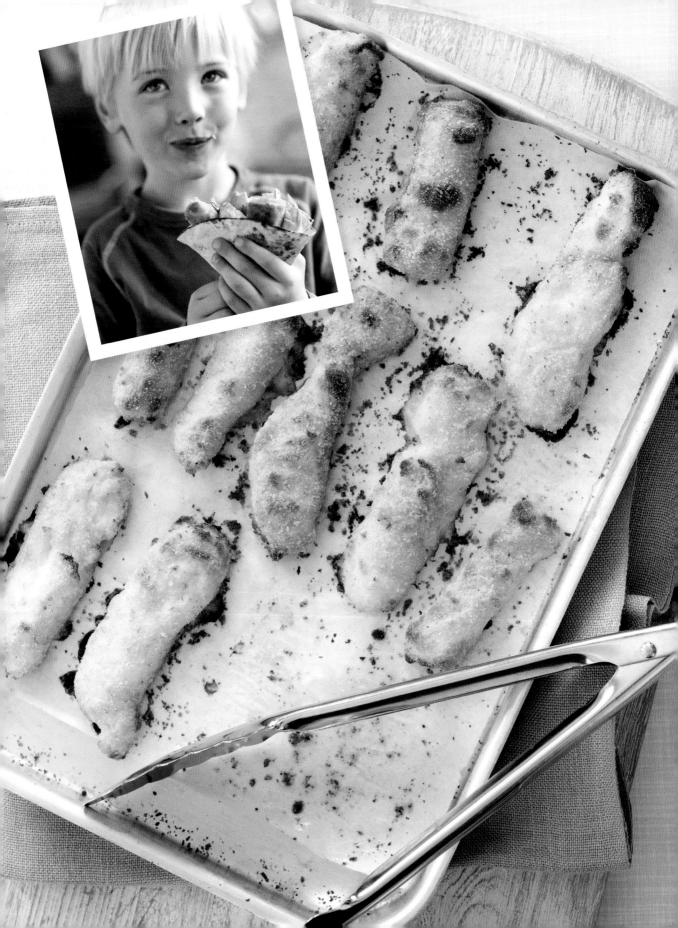

When the kids are STARRRRVING and you need something quick, these sauces are lifesavers. There's no need to be too specific about quantities. They are guidelines to help you to please grumbling tummies.

Very, Very, Very Quick Pasta Dishes

EACH SAUCE MAKES 2 adult or 4 kid-sized portions
PREPARATION TIME 5 minutes
COOKING TIME 10 minutes

SMOKED SALMON, CREAM CHEESE AND CHIVE FARFALLE

250g/9oz/2¾ cups farfalle
250g/9oz cream cheese
5 tbsp milk
4 ripe tomatoes, deseeded and diced
175g/6oz smoked salmon, cut into
   small pieces
1 handful of chives, finely chopped

1 Bring a pan of water to the boil, add the pasta and return to the boil. Simmer for about 10 minutes until just tender. Drain well, then return the pasta to the hot pan.

2 Meanwhile, put the cream cheese and milk into a small pan and heat gently, stirring until melted. Add the tomatoes and stir for about 1 minute, then stir in the smoked salmon and chives. Pour the sauce over the drained pasta and stir together. Serve hot.

SAUSAGE, PESTO AND TOMATO PENNE

a drizzle of olive oil
4 sausages, skinned and broken into
   chunks
400g/14oz/1¾ cups canned chopped
   tomatoes
2 tbsp pesto sauce
4 tbsp cream cheese (optional)
250g/9oz/2¾ cups penne

1 Heat the oil in a small pan over a medium heat, add the sausage chunks and fry for 5 minutes until cooked and becoming golden, breaking down the meat with a wooden spoon. Stir in the tomatoes, bring to a simmer, then cook for 5 minutes. Stir in the pesto. Stir in the cream cheese, if you like, for a creamier sauce.

2 Meanwhile, bring a pan of water to the boil, add the pasta and return to the boil. Simmer for about 10 minutes until just tender. Drain well, then return to the hot pan. Pour the sauce over the drained pasta and stir together. Serve hot.

CREAMY PEA, BASIL AND HAM LINGUINE

250g/9oz linguine
250g/9oz mascarpone or cream cheese
2 tbsp milk
3 tbsp tomato or sun-dried tomato
  purée/paste
1 large handful of frozen peas
1 small handful of basil leaves, chopped
4 slices of ham, finely chopped
sea salt and freshly ground black pepper

1 Bring a pan of water to the boil, add the pasta and return to the boil. Simmer for about 10 minutes until just tender. Drain well, then return the pasta to the hot pan.

2 Meanwhile, put the mascarpone, milk and tomato purée/paste in a saucepan over a low heat and stir until the cheese has melted. Add the peas, basil and ham and stir for 2 minutes until heated through. Season lightly with salt and pepper. Pour the sauce over the drained pasta and stir together. Serve hot.

BUTTERY MUSHROOM AND PARMESAN FUSILLI

250g/9oz/2¾ cups fusilli
50g/1¾oz butter
200g/7oz button or baby chestnut
  mushrooms, sliced
2 garlic cloves, crushed
juice of 1 small lemon
2 tbsp chopped basil or parsley leaves
  (optional)
50g/1¾oz/⅔ cup freshly grated
  Parmesan cheese
a splash of double/heavy cream
  (optional)

1 Bring a pan of water to the boil, add the pasta and return to the boil. Simmer for about 10 minutes until just tender. Drain well, then return the pasta to the hot pan.

2 Meanwhile, melt the butter in a small frying pan over a medium heat and add the mushrooms. Cook for a few minutes until they are softened and starting to become golden. Add the garlic and lemon juice, and the basil, if using, and cook for a further 2 minutes. Spoon the sauce over the drained pasta, sprinkle with the Parmesan and stir together. For an extra creamy finish you can add a splash of double/heavy cream, if you like. Serve hot.

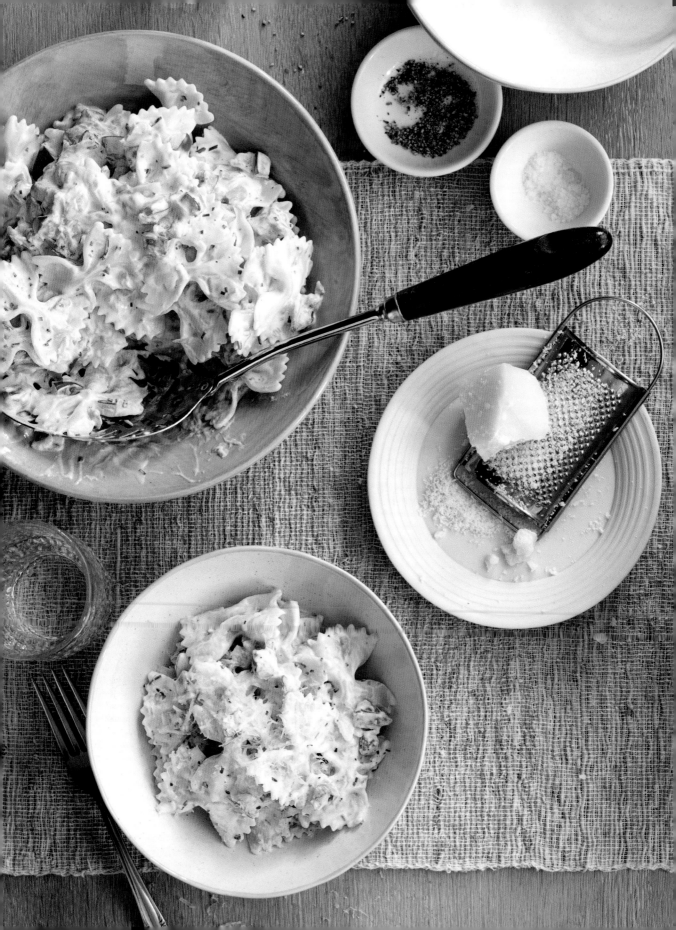

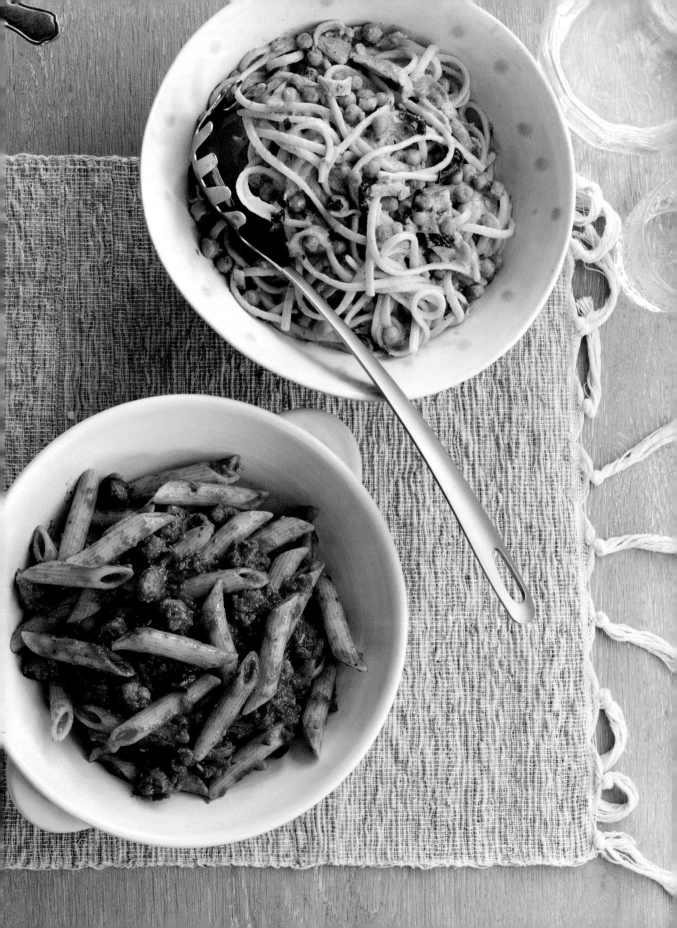

Always, always have these ingredients in your cupboard and you will never be without a delicious evening meal. Apart from the onion, everything comes in a packet, jar or can and lasts for ages. If you don't have anchovies, adding a can of flaked tuna makes a tasty substitute.

Pantry Pasta Puttanesca

MAKES 2 adult or 4 kid-sized portions
PREPARATION TIME 15 minutes
COOKING TIME 15 minutes

2 tbsp olive oil
1 onion, finely diced
½ red chilli, deseeded (or seeds left in for a spicier finish) and finely sliced or ¼ tsp dried chilli/hot pepper flakes
4 anchovy fillets, finely chopped
400g/14oz/1¾ cups canned chopped tomatoes
½ tsp dried oregano
180g/6¼oz/1½ cups black kalamata olives, halved and pitted
1 tbsp capers, chopped if large
250g/9oz/2¾ cups pasta, such as penne
freshly grated Parmesan cheese, for sprinkling
sea salt and freshly ground black pepper

1 Heat the oil in a large frying pan over a medium heat, add the onion and chilli and fry for about 5 minutes until the onion is soft but not coloured. Add the anchovies and cook for a further couple of minutes, stirring all the time. Stir in the tomatoes, oregano, olives and capers. Bring to the boil and season lightly with salt and pepper, then reduce the heat to low and leave to simmer for 8–10 minutes.

2 Meanwhile, bring a pan of lightly salted water to the boil, add the pasta and return to the boil. Simmer for about 10 minutes until just tender. Drain well.

3 Add the pasta to the sauce and stir well. Serve sprinkled with plenty of Parmesan cheese.

Lifesaver for handy dinners
storing the puttanesca sauce in jars

If you have the ingredients, it's a real lifesaver if you make double (or more) and store it in jars to use when needed. All you need to do is divide the cooked sauce into hot, sterilized jars and seal loosely with a lid. Put them in a roasting pan lined with a folded dish towel and fill 2cm/¾in deep with hot water. Put in a preheated oven at 160°C/315°F/gas 2–3 for 25 minutes, then carefully remove from the pan and seal tightly. Store in a cool, dark place and use within 6 months. Once open, store in the refrigerator and use within a few days.

A really simple recipe that you could call Asian Prawn Noodle Broth if you fancy giving it a posh name. This is a perfect dish to make for kids as well as adults. It's almost as easy as making a shop-bought pot. Just make sure you go careful on the chilli (as they vary so much) if you are intending to serve it to your kids.

Posh Pot Noodle

MAKES 2 adult or 4 kid-sized portions
PREPARATION TIME 5 minutes
COOKING TIME 10 minutes

600ml/21fl oz/scant 2½ cups very hot chicken or vegetable stock or miso soup
150g/5½oz dried udon, rice or egg noodles
2.5cm/1in piece of root ginger, peeled and finely grated
1 long red chilli, very thinly sliced (deseeded if you want a less fiery flavour)
2 large handfuls of raw, peeled king prawns/jumbo shrimp, fresh or frozen, defrosted
2 handfuls of vegetables, such as sugarsnap peas, baby corn or asparagus
1½ tbsp soft light brown sugar
1½ tbsp fish sauce
4 spring onions/scallions, very finely sliced (optional)
juice of 1 lime
2 large handfuls of coriander/cilantro and/or mint leaves

1 Put the stock in a saucepan over a medium heat and bring to the boil. Add the noodles, ginger and chilli, reduce the heat to low and simmer for about 3 minutes until the noodles are beginning to soften.

2 Add the prawns/shrimp, vegetables, sugar and fish sauce. Cook for a few minutes until the prawns/shrimp and vegetables are cooked through.

3 Stir in the spring onions/scallions, if using, the lime juice and herbs. Serve hot.

Leftovers are lovely jazzed up

nutty noodles
If you don't use the whole pack of noodles, they make a great quick lunch when you are on your own (or double up if you are not). Cook **1 portion of udon, rice** or **egg noodles** according to the packet instructions. Drain and toss with **a drizzle of chilli** or **sesame oil**, **1 tbsp oyster sauce**, **2 thinly sliced spring onions/scallions**, **a squeeze of lime juice** or **a splash of rice vinegar** and **1 small handful of chopped coriander/cilantro leaves**. Scatter over **2 tbsp chopped roasted peanuts** or **cashew nuts** and serve.

Having a packet of gnocchi in the refrigerator is a really good idea. It's a nice alternative to pasta and pretty much goes with anything. I'm always trying out different combos with stuff that I find in my refrigerator. The recipe below has become a household favourite. Once you get the hang of this recipe, experiment with your own ideas – why not try swapping the broccoli for that bag of spinach you always buy but rarely use.

Broccoli, Mushroom and Parmesan Gnocchi

MAKES 2 adult or 4 kid-sized portions
PREPARATION TIME 10 minutes
COOKING TIME 12 minutes

350–500g/12oz–1lb 2oz shop-bought gnocchi (depending on how hungry you are)
2 tbsp olive oil
150g/5½oz mushrooms, quartered or thickly sliced
150g/5½oz broccoli, broken into small florets
2 garlic cloves, crushed
2 tbsp water or white wine (optional)
4 tbsp double/heavy or single/light cream
¼ tsp freshly grated nutmeg
a good squeeze of lemon juice
25g/1oz/¼ cup freshly grated Parmesan cheese
sea salt and freshly ground black pepper

1 Bring a pan of lightly salted water to the boil, add the gnocchi and return to the boil. Cook for 2 minutes, then drain well.

2 Heat the oil in a large saucepan over a medium heat, add the mushrooms, broccoli and garlic and cook for 5–6 minutes until they are tender. If they start to stick to the pan or to go brown, add a splash of water or white wine, if you have some open, to create a little steam. Add the cooked gnocchi and fry for 2 minutes, then add the cream and bring to a bubble.

3 Add the nutmeg, lemon juice and Parmesan, and season lightly with salt and pepper. Stir the ingredients together for a couple of minutes until well mixed. Serve hot.

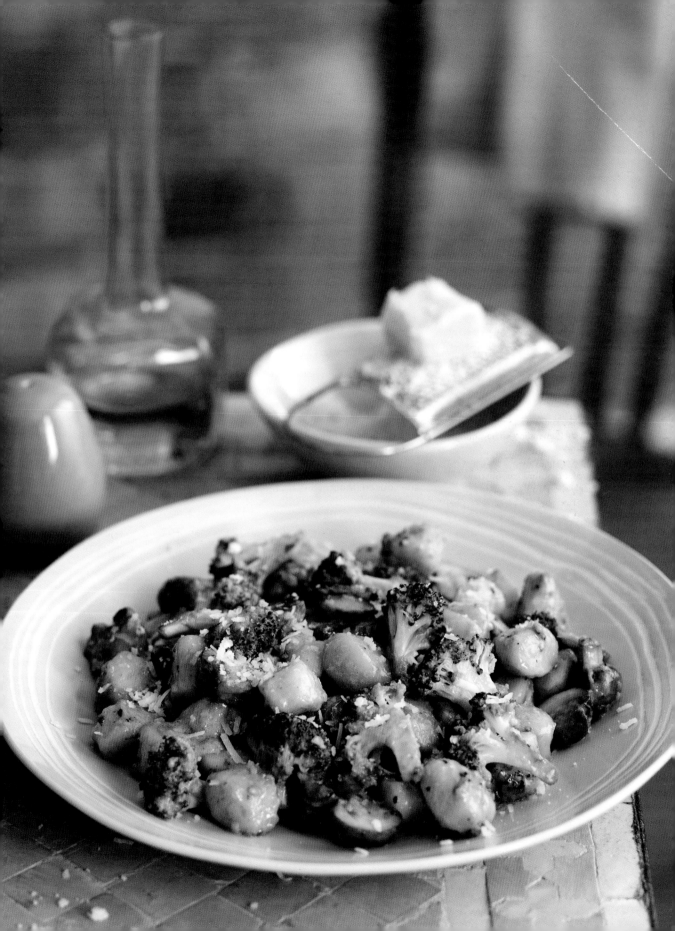

I always get posh cheese in when we have friends round for dinner, then find it is only rarely eaten (partly due to my friends having to get back to relieve their babysitters), so I concocted this deliciously filling recipe to use up some of that cheese.

Lemon Linguine with Walnuts, Spinach and Blue Cheese

MAKES 2 adult or 4 kid-sized portions
PREPARATION TIME 10 minutes
COOKING TIME 12 minutes

250g/9oz linguine
50g/1¾oz/½ cup walnut pieces
1 tbsp olive oil
1 red onion, finely sliced
finely grated zest and juice of 1 lemon
200g/7oz/1¼ cups frozen spinach, defrosted
150g/5½oz blue cheese, such as Gorgonzola, dolcelatte, Danish blue or Stilton, cut into cubes
1 tbsp extra virgin olive oil
sea salt and freshly ground black pepper

1 Bring a pan of lightly salted water to the boil, add the linguine and return to the boil. Simmer for about 10 minutes until just tender. Drain, reserving 2 tbsp of the cooking water.

2 Meanwhile, heat a frying pan over a medium heat, add the walnuts and toast for a few minutes until they colour slightly, tossing the pan gently. Tip into a bowl.

3 Return the pan to the heat and add the olive oil. Add the onion and fry gently for a few minutes until softened and golden. Stir in the lemon zest and juice and the reserved pasta water and bring to the boil. Add the linguine and stir into the lemony juices for about 1 minute. Add the spinach leaves, the diced blue cheese, toasted walnuts and a good twist of black pepper. (Salt shouldn't be necessary as the cheese is naturally salty.) Toss together until everything is well combined and the cheese is beginning to melt.

4 Drizzle over the extra virgin olive oil and serve hot.

Leftovers for a teatime treat
walnut and honey butter
Use the rest of the packet of walnuts to make this delicious butter. Lightly toast **50g/1¾oz/½ cup walnuts** until golden. Leave to cool, then pop into a small blender and whizz together with **100g/3½oz butter**, **a pinch of ground cinnamon** and **3 tbsp clear honey**. Use to spread over toast, warm baguettes or crumpets, or to melt over the top of pancakes.

This is a lifesaver for when you can't be bothered to make much of an effort or you think you are out of provisions. When that happens, check your store cupboard and refrigerator and you might be surprised. These are just suggestions for what you could do, but generally if you have some onion, oil, beans and tomatoes as a base, you can add an array of ingredients depending on what you can find. This is perfect for two served with baked potatoes or on its own makes a hearty meal for one. If you also have some chorizo or bacon in the refrigerator, fry it with the onions. A handful of fresh or frozen spinach could be stirred through at the end, or some chopped coriander/cilantro, basil or parsley leaves.

Store Cupboard Bean and Tomato Stew with Baked Potatoes

MAKES 2 adult or 4 kid-sized portions
PREPARATION TIME 5 minutes
COOKING TIME 20 minutes

2 potatoes
1 tbsp olive oil
½ white or red onion, sliced
1 garlic clove, crushed
125ml/4fl oz/½ cup white wine, red wine, sherry or beer (depending on what's open)
240g/8½oz canned chickpeas/garbanzos or cannellini, borlotti, kidney, mixed or butter beans, drained, or even baked beans, rinsed of their juice
400g/14oz/1¾ cups canned chopped tomatoes
1 bottled or canned roasted red pepper, sliced
1 handful of black or green olives, pitted
a pinch of dried chilli/hot pepper flakes or chilli powder
sea salt and freshly ground black pepper
2 tbsp butter, to serve

1 Preheat the oven to 220°C/425°F/gas 7.

2 Prick the potatoes a few times with a fork. Microwave on High for 5 minutes until soft, then transfer to the oven to crisp the skins.

3 Meanwhile, heat the oil in a frying pan over a low heat and fry the onion and garlic for a few minutes until softened. Add the wine, sherry or beer. Bring to the boil, then reduce the heat and simmer for about 5 minutes to cook away any alcohol (making this fine for the kids) and to reduce the quantity by half.

4 Stir in all the remaining ingredients and season lightly with salt and pepper. Bring to a simmer, then cook for 5–8 minutes until the tomatoes have thickened.

5 Split open the potatoes, mix in the butter, then serve topped with the bean and tomato stew.

Serve these on their own as a snack or with tomato salsa and a rocket/ arugula and avocado salad. A chunk of garlic bread on the side goes nicely too. For added flexibility, once you have done your prep you can cook the fritters as and when you need them. The mixture will keep in the refrigerator for a good few hours.

Ricotta and Courgette Fritters

MAKES 2 adult or 4 kid-sized portions
PREPARATION TIME 10 minutes
COOKING TIME 8 minutes each

250g/9oz ricotta cheese
2 courgettes/zucchini, grated
50g/1¾oz/⅓ cup peas or sweetcorn
75g/2½oz/scant ⅔ cup self-raising flour
½ tsp paprika
1½ tbsp chopped mint or basil leaves or chives
finely grated zest of 1 small lemon
2 eggs, lightly beaten
olive oil, for frying
sea salt and freshly ground black pepper (optional)

1 Mix together the ricotta, courgettes/zucchini, peas, flour, paprika, herbs, lemon zest and eggs. Season lightly with salt and pepper, if using. (The mixture can be kept in the refrigerator for a few hours or cooked straight away.)

2 Heat about 1cm/½in of oil in a frying pan over a medium heat, add tablespoonfuls of the mixture and cook for 3–4 minutes on each side until golden and firm to touch. This should make 12 fritters so you may need to cook them in batches and keep the first ones warm while you continue to cook the remaining fritters.

3 Serve hot.

Lifesaver for pasta

pea pesto

It's worth defrosting some extra peas when making the fritters so you can whizz up a vibrant, nutritious pesto to toss into pasta for another day. This makes plenty for 2 adult and 2 kid-sized portions. Put **200g/7oz/1¼ cups defrosted frozen peas** in a food processor bowl along with **50g/1¾oz/⅓ cup lightly toasted pine nuts**, **1 garlic clove**, **1 large handful of chopped basil leaves**, **½ small handful of chopped mint leaves**, **50g/1¾oz/⅔ cup freshly grated Parmesan cheese**, **125ml/4fl oz/½ cup olive oil** and a little **sea salt** and **freshly ground black pepper**. Blend until smooth, adding a little water if the pesto seems too thick. Transfer to a bowl and cover with a thin layer of **oil** to help prevent discolouring. Use within 3 days. The pesto will thicken in the refrigerator so, when using, toss **1–2 tbsp pasta cooking water** in with the pesto and pasta to loosen it.

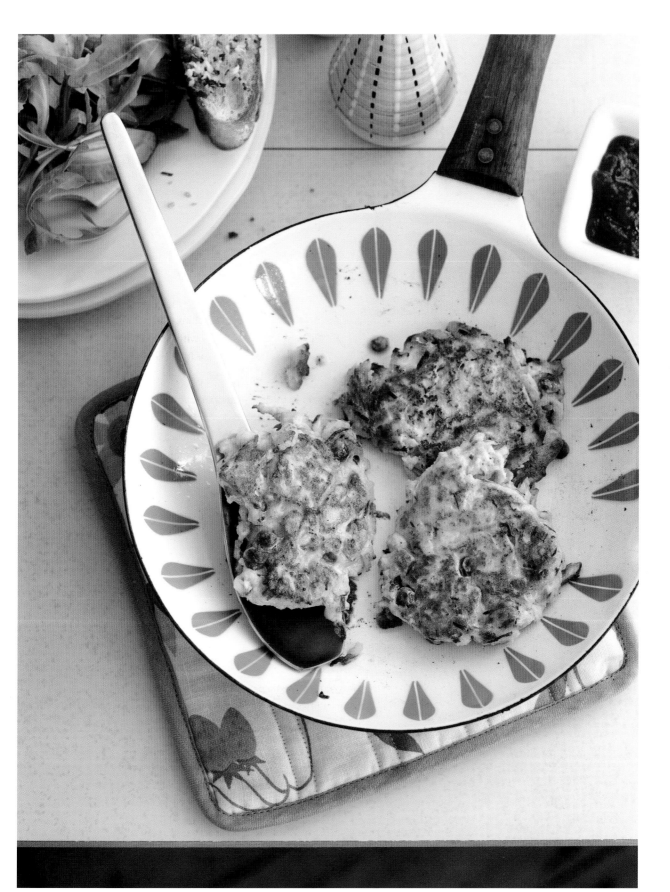

Stir-fries are the ultimate fast food, great for busy families, and most fish, meat and vegetable stir-fry combinations can be lifted with a sauce. These recipes can be made ahead and stored in a jar or sealed container and used as and when you like (they'll keep in the refrigerator for a week or so) so I've increased the serving quantities. Simply add to the stir-fry at the last minute to heat through.

Stir Crazy

EACH SAUCE MAKES 4 adult or 8 kid-sized portions
PREPARATION TIME 10 minutes
COOKING TIME 8 minutes

SWEET AND SOUR PINEAPPLE SAUCE

200ml/7fl oz/scant 1 cup pineapple juice
1 tbsp cornflour/cornstarch
1 tbsp soy sauce
1 tbsp rice vinegar or white wine vinegar
1 tbsp tomato purée/paste

1 Mix a little of the pineapple juice into the cornflour/cornstarch to make a paste, then simply put all the ingredients into a small saucepan. Put over a medium heat and bring to the boil, stirring occasionally, then reduce the heat and leave to simmer for 1–2 minutes.

2 Stir into a stir-fry dish for the last minute to heat through.

COCONUT AND PEANUT SATAY SAUCE

a drizzle of sunflower oil
2 garlic cloves, crushed
200ml/7fl oz/scant 1 cup canned coconut milk
2 tbsp peanut butter (crunchy or smooth)
1 tsp soy sauce
a pinch of dried chilli/hot pepper flakes
a squeeze of lime juice

1 Heat the oil in a saucepan over a low heat, add the garlic and fry for a few minutes until softened but not coloured. Add the remaining ingredients, bring to the boil, then reduce the heat and leave to simmer for 3–4 minutes.

2 Stir into a stir-fry dish at the last minute to heat through.

OYSTER, SPRING ONION AND GINGER SAUCE

2 tbsp sesame oil
5cm/2in piece of root ginger, peeled and finely chopped or grated
2 garlic cloves, crushed
4 spring onions/scallions, chopped
4 tbsp oyster sauce
6 tbsp orange juice
1 tsp rice vinegar or white wine vinegar

1 Heat the oil in a small saucepan, add the ginger, garlic and spring onions/scallions and cook gently for about 5 minutes. Add the remaining ingredients, bring to the boil, then reduce the heat and leave to simmer for 2–3 minutes.

2 Stir into a stir-fry dish at the last minute to heat through.

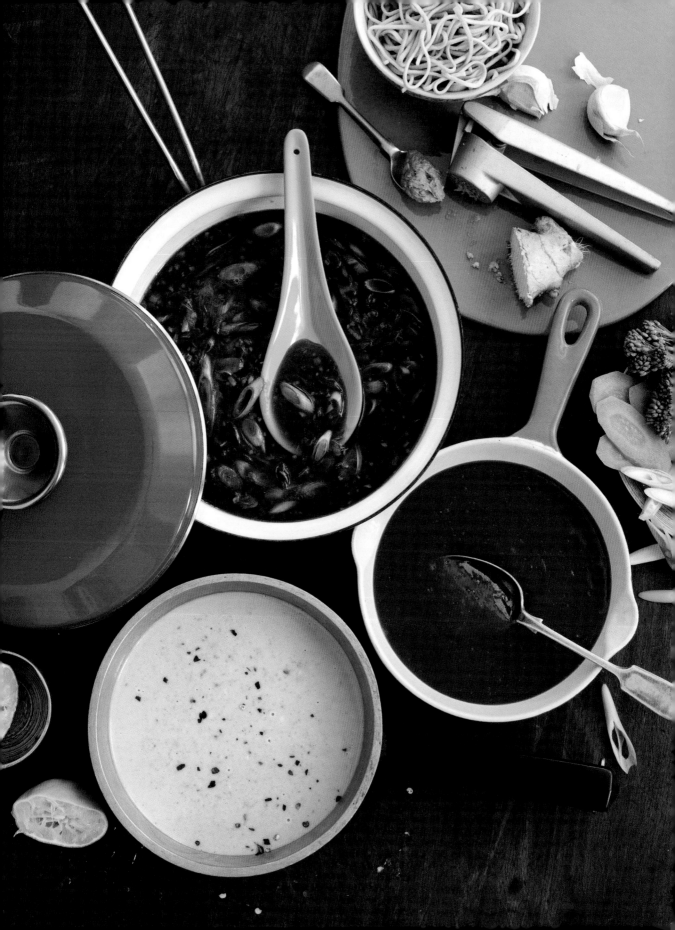

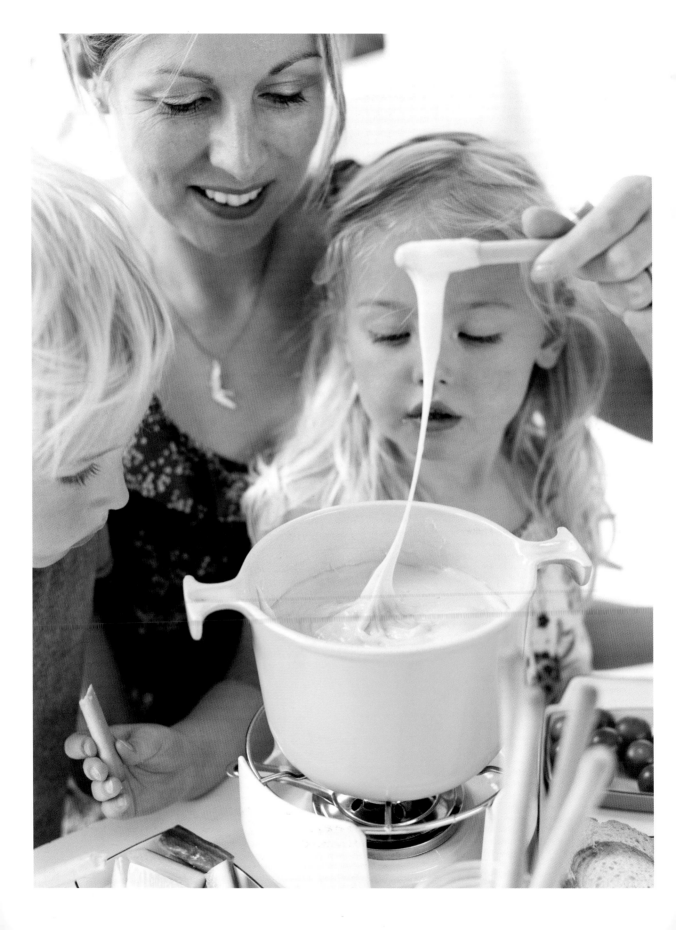

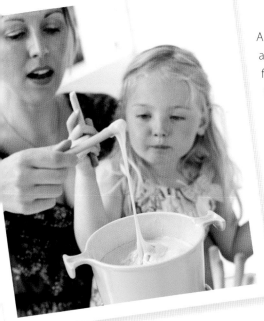

A great recipe for your kids to make at home or for entertaining a group of kids, you can dip just about anything in this delicious fondue (although maybe avoid toy cars and Barbie dolls!). To save time, buy bags of ready-grated cheese, and for a more grown-up version, use wine instead of apple juice.

Under 18 and Over 18 Cheese Fondue

MAKES 2 adult or 4 kid-sized portions
PREPARATION TIME 10 minutes
COOKING TIME 5 minutes

FOR THE CHEESE FONDUE
100ml/3½fl oz/scant ½ cup apple juice
   or white wine
2 tsp cornflour/cornstarch
1 small garlic clove, halved
100g/3½oz/scant ⅔ cup grated
   Emmental or Gruyère cheese
100g/3½oz/scant ⅔ cup grated Cheddar
   cheese
¼ tsp freshly grated nutmeg

FOR DIPPING
you choose – virtually anything goes:
• cubes of crusty bread or breadsticks
• lightly cooked vegetables, such as
   broccoli, cauliflower, courgette/
   zucchini or baby corn
• sticks of carrot, cucumber, pepper or
   cherry tomatoes
• grapes, sliced apple or pear
• cooked tortellini or other small filled
   pasta shapes

1 Mix 2 tbsp of the apple juice into the cornflour/cornstarch to make a paste. Pour the remaining apple juice into a saucepan and add the garlic. Bring to a simmer over a low heat, without allowing it to boil. Gradually stir in the cheese, allowing it to melt, then stir in the cornflour/cornstarch paste. Cook for a couple of minutes until it is silky smooth and thickened, stirring all the time. If you can find it, fish out the garlic clove, then finish by stirring in the nutmeg.

2 If you know it will be eaten quickly, simply pour the fondue into a warm bowl, or you can, of course, be more traditional and serve in a fondue pot – just make sure kids are careful with the open flame. Or, if you have one, it can be served in a slow cooker set on low.

Leftovers for a family favourite
cauliflower mac 'n' cheese
Warm any leftover cheese fondue with **a little milk** to loosen, then stir in the same quantity of **cooked mashed or puréed cauliflower**. Mix into **cooked macaroni** – you'll need about twice as much macaroni as cauliflower – scatter with a little **grated Cheddar cheese** and grill/broil until bubbling.

I have been cooking versions of this recipe for years as it is so simple and flavoursome. It's great for throwing in the oven and tucking into with a green salad, ciabatta and a glass of wine. Kids love the flavours too. For them, I just chop the cooked chicken into smaller pieces, and often use half wine and half stock. It freezes well and any left over makes a great lifesaver meal for another day.

Mediterranean Baked Chicken and Rice

MAKES 2 adult and 4 kid-sized portions
PREPARATION TIME 15 minutes
COOKING TIME 45 minutes

4 skinless chicken breasts
2 tbsp olive oil
1 white or red onion, chopped
75g/2½oz piece of chorizo, diced (optional)
1 red pepper, deseeded and thinly sliced
2 garlic cloves, crushed
250g/9oz/1¼ cups long-grain rice
500ml/17fl oz/2 cups passata/Italian sieved tomatoes
375ml/13fl oz/1½ cups white wine or chicken stock
1 tsp balsamic vinegar
8–10 sun-dried tomatoes, roughly chopped
180g/6¼oz/1½ cups black or green olives, halved and pitted
1 handful of basil leaves, chopped
sea salt and freshly ground black pepper

1 Preheat the oven to 180°C/350°F/gas 4.

2 Cut 2–3 deep slits in the chicken breasts and season lightly with salt and pepper. Heat the oil in a flameproof casserole dish, add the chicken and fry over a high heat for a couple of minutes on each side until brown. Remove the chicken from the dish.

3 Add the onion, chorizo, if using, red pepper and garlic and fry over a medium heat for 5 minutes until the onion is softened. Stir in the rice and, when it is coated in the oil, add the remaining ingredients. Season lightly with salt and pepper and bring to a simmer.

4 Return the chicken and any juices to the dish, pushing each piece into the sauce so it is partly covered. Cover with a lid and bake for 35 minutes until the chicken is cooked through and the sauce is rich, juicy and tasty. Serve hot.

Leftovers for a salad
chicken rice salad

You can freeze individual portions of this recipe, then defrost and reheat thoroughly within 3 months, or why not try this delicious salad. Put any leftovers in the refrigerator as soon as possible. The next day, cut up any **chicken** into smaller pieces and stir into some **cooked rice** with some **olive oil** and **balsamic vinegar**. Toss in some **salad leaves**, **diced cucumber** and **radishes** and some **sliced or diced avocado** to create a delicious salad.

This recipe ticks a lot of boxes: it can be frozen; it can feed the kids, then the grown-ups; it's a lovely family meal; it can even be taken next door as a 'welcome to the neighbourhood' gift; and it can be served with pasta, baked or mashed potatoes, rice or couscous. It's more versatile than a Swiss Army knife! This is another recipe that is worth making in a bigger quantity to make Sausage Pot Pies (below) or to freeze.

Yummy Sausage Pot

MAKES 2 adult and 4 kid-sized portions
PREPARATION TIME 15 minutes
COOKING TIME 45 minutes

2 tbsp olive oil
8–12 pork sausages, left whole or cut into smaller pieces
1 onion, sliced or chopped
2 garlic cloves, crushed
1 red pepper, deseeded and sliced or chopped
1 large carrot, peeled and grated
100g/3½oz mushrooms, chopped
650ml/22½fl oz/scant 2¾ cups passata/ Italian sieved tomatoes
a pinch of dried mixed herbs
1 tsp caster/superfine sugar
1 tsp balsamic vinegar
sea salt and freshly ground black pepper

1 Heat the oil in a large saucepan or flameproof casserole, add the sausages and fry over a medium-high heat for about 10 minutes until golden brown.

2 Add the onion, garlic and red pepper, reduce the heat and fry for about 5 minutes until the vegetables are beginning to soften. Stir in the carrot and mushrooms and fry for a couple of minutes before adding the remaining ingredients. Bring to the boil, then reduce the heat, cover loosely with a lid and leave to simmer for about 30 minutes until all the ingredients are cooked through and the sauce is thick. Season lightly with salt and pepper. (Anything not eaten straight away will keep in the refrigerator for a couple of days or can be frozen for up to 3 months, or why not try my Sausage Pot Pies, below).

3 Serve hot.

Leftovers for family pies
sausage pot pies

Spoon the Yummy Sausage Pot into a pie dish or smaller dishes. If you don't have a huge amount left over, then bulk it out by mixing in some **drained canned cannellini** or **butter beans**. Top the mixture with rolled out **puff** or **shortcrust pastry**. Pierce a small hole in the top to let steam escape. Make an egg wash by mixing **1 egg yolk** with **1 tbsp water** and brush it over the pastry, or use **oil** or **milk**. Bake in a preheated oven at 200°C/400°F/gas 6 for about 20–30 minutes until the pastry is golden.

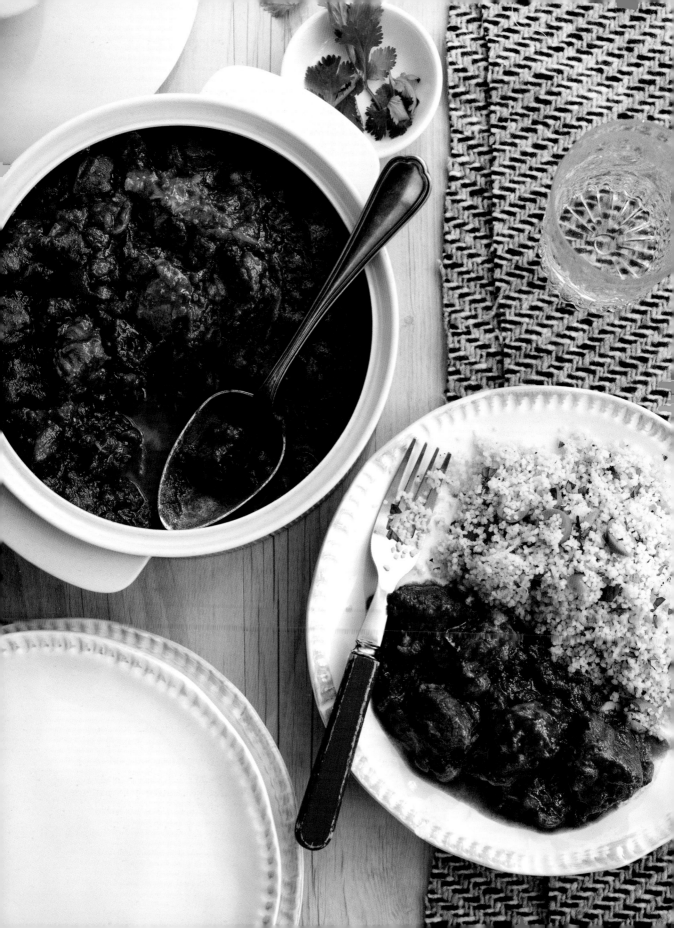

Kids will love the sweetness coming from the apricots and the aromatic cinnamon in this stew. For an authentic touch, serve it with plain couscous, or you can flavour the couscous with a little chopped mint, grated lemon zest and sliced green olives and serve it to friends as a dinner party main course. If you have any leftovers, you can make a Moroccan Shepherd's Pie (see below).

Moroccan Lamb Stew

MAKES 2 adult and 4 kid-sized portions
PREPARATION TIME 10 minutes
COOKING TIME 1½ hours

1 tbsp olive oil
1 onion, thinly sliced
750g/1lb 10oz diced lamb shoulder
2 tsp ground coriander
2 tsp hot paprika
3 tsp ground cinnamon
800g/1lb 12oz/3½ cups canned chopped tomatoes
150g/5½oz/1¼ cups sultanas/golden raisins or chopped apricots
1 handful of coriander/cilantro leaves, chopped
sea salt and freshly ground black pepper
couscous, to serve

1 Heat the oil in a flameproof casserole dish over a medium heat, add the onion and fry for a few minutes until starting to soften. Increase the heat to high, add the lamb and cook for a few minutes until browned, stirring continuously.

2 Add the spices, season to taste with salt and pepper and cook for about 1 minute, stirring. Add the tomatoes and 200ml/7fl oz/scant 1 cup water. Bring to the boil, then reduce the heat to low, cover with a lid and leave to simmer for 1 hour, stirring a couple of times during cooking.

3 After 1 hour, remove the lid, add the sultanas/golden raisins and cook for a further 20–30 minutes until the lamb is tender. (The dish can easily be frozen at this point for up to 3 months. Or you could make a Moroccan Shepherd's Pie out of any leftovers – see below).

4 Scatter with the coriander/cilantro leaves and serve with couscous.

Leftovers for a taste of Morocco
moroccan shepherd's pie
Simply spoon any leftover **lamb** into an ovenproof dish and stir in some **frozen peas**, **green beans** or **broad/fava beans**. Top with **mashed sweet potato** or a combination of **carrots** and **white potatoes**. Dot with **butter** and bake in a preheated oven at 200°C/400°F/gas 6 for 20–30 minutes until the filling is hot and the topping is golden.

Here's an alternative recipe for that minced/ground meat we all buy every week without fail or that we have kicking about in the freezer. Come rain or shine, this will please all the family with the rich delicious flavours in both the sauce and meatballs. It freezes well so I make extra.

Meatballs with Olives

MAKES 2 adult and 4 kid-sized portions
PREPARATION TIME 15 minutes, plus
   10 minutes chilling (optional)
COOKING TIME 55 minutes

500g/1lb 2oz minced/ground meat,
   such as beef, pork or lamb
1 onion, roughly chopped
2 garlic cloves, roughly chopped
1 egg, lightly beaten
2 tbsp chopped mint leaves or 1 tsp
   dried mint
¼ tsp freshly grated nutmeg
3 tbsp olive oil
1 large aubergine/eggplant, finely diced
   into small pieces
400g/14oz/1¾ cups canned chopped
   tomatoes
80ml/2½fl oz/⅓ cup red wine, water or
   stock
1 tbsp red wine vinegar
1 tsp dried oregano
¼ tsp ground cinnamon
2 handfuls of black olives, pitted and
   chopped
sea salt and freshly ground black pepper

TO SERVE
4 tbsp natural or Greek yogurt
cooked rice or pitta breads

1 Put the minced/ground meat, onion, garlic, egg, mint and nutmeg in a food processor and season lightly with salt and pepper. Process until thoroughly combined.

2 Using wet hands to stop the mixture sticking to you, shape the meatball mixture into balls the about size of a whole walnut in its shell. If you have the time, pop them in the freezer for 10 minutes to firm up. (Alternatively, you can make the meatballs up to a day in advance and keep them in the refrigerator until you are ready to cook.)

3 Heat the oil in a large, shallow pan over a medium-high heat, add the meatballs and fry for a few minutes until they start to colour, then remove them from the pan. Add the aubergine/eggplant and fry for a couple of minutes. Stir in the tomatoes, then the wine and wine vinegar. Add the oregano, cinnamon and olives, season lightly with salt and pepper and bring to the boil. Pop in the meatballs, reduce the heat, cover with a lid and leave to simmer gently for 45 minutes until the sauce has thickened and the meatballs are cooked through.

4 Drizzle over a spoonful of natural or Greek yogurt and serve with cooked rice or pitta breads.

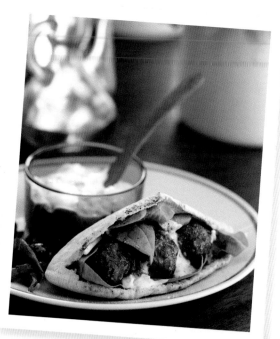

Leftovers for Greek-style lunch
meatball and tzatziki pittas
For a simple lunch, warm and split some **pitta bread**, then fill with leftover **meatballs** (without too much sauce), either heated through or cold. Add **a few baby spinach leaves**, **a dollop of tzatziki** and some **pickled chillies** and tuck in.

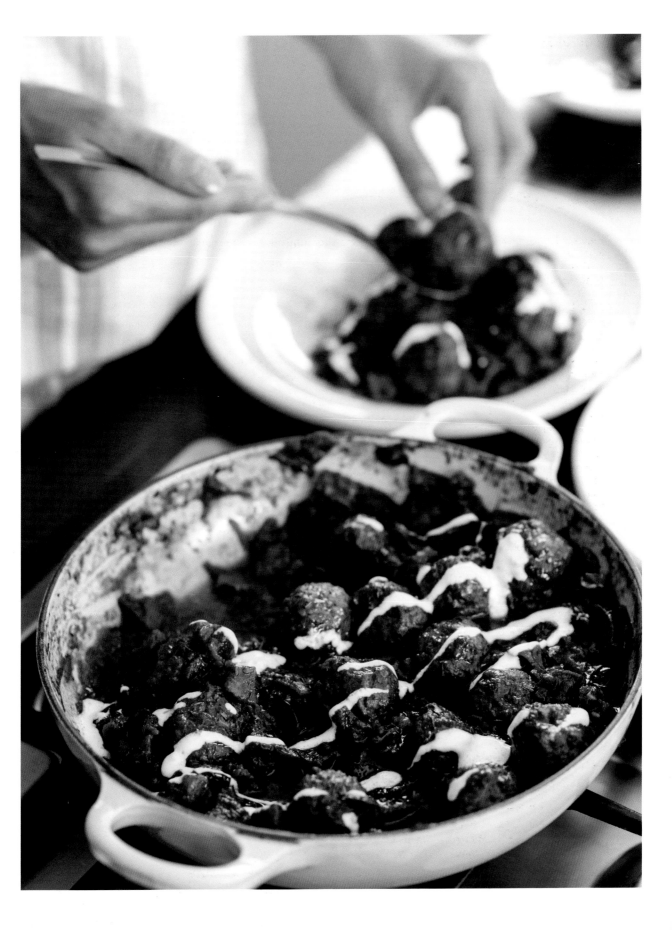

Bolognese sauce is such a household favourite, and whenever I make it, I always make plenty and freeze some for when I need a ready-prepared dinner for the family – all I need to do is boil up some pasta. This is really a useful standby as you can serve it with rice or baked potato as well as pasta, make it into lasagne, cannelloni or shepherd's pie, or use it to fill pancakes or tortillas.

Good All-round Bolognese

MAKES 6 adult and 6 kid-sized portions
PREPARATION TIME 10 minutes using pre-
   made Vegetable Starter Mix or
   20 minutes from scratch
COOKING TIME 1¾ hours

2 tbsp olive oil
½ recipe quantity Vegetable Starter Mix
   (see below)
1kg/2lb 4oz minced/ground beef
250ml/9fl oz/1 cup red wine
1 beef stock cube or 1 tbsp concentrated
   beef stock
1 tbsp chopped oregano leaves or mixed
   herbs
750g/1lb 10oz/3 cups canned chopped
   tomatoes
2 tbsp tomato purée/paste
1 tsp caster/superfine sugar
1 tsp balsamic vinegar
75g/2½ oz/scant 1 cup freshly grated
   Parmesan cheese
sea salt and freshly ground black pepper

FOR THE PASTA
about 100g/3½oz/heaped 1 cup dried
   pasta per person

1 Heat the oil in a large pan over a medium heat, add the starter mix and fry for 5 minutes until the vegetables are starting to brown. Stir in the minced/ground beef, breaking it down with a wooden spoon so you don't have any large clumps. Cook over a high heat until browned. Pour in the wine and boil for 2 minutes, then add the remaining ingredients except the Parmesan. Season lightly with salt and pepper.

2 Cover loosely with a lid and cook over a low heat for about 1½ hours, or longer if preferred, until the sauce is rich and thick. (Alternatively, you can cook the sauce in a preheated oven at 180°C/350°F/gas 4 for the same length of time.) Leave the sauce to rest for 10 minutes. (Any sauce you are not serving can be left to cool, then divided into portions to store in the refrigerator for up to 3 days or in the freezer for up to 3 months.)

3 While the sauce is resting, bring a large pan of lightly salted water to the boil, add the pasta and return to the boil. Simmer for about 10 minutes until just tender. Drain well.

4 Sprinkle the bolognese with the Parmesan and serve with the pasta.

Lifesaver for the freezer
vegetable starter mix – soffrito

This is brilliant for using a glut of vegetables and makes a mega-convenient standby. It's based on the Italian *soffrito*: finely chopped aromatic ingredients softly fried and used as a base for soups, casseroles, tomato sauces, bolognese, chilli or shepherd's pie, to name just a few. Use these quantities as a guide: **2 large onions, 2 large carrots, 2 deseeded red peppers, 2 courgettes/zucchini, 8 garlic cloves, 4 celery stalks, 150g/5½oz mushrooms** (optional) and **4 tbsp olive oil**. Finely chop the vegetables (I use a food processor) and fry in the olive oil until soft but not coloured. If you get a lot of water coming out of them, just increase the heat so it evaporates off. Either use some or all of the vegetables straight away to start off a dish, or remove from the heat, cool, then divide up, label and store in the refrigerator for up to 3 days or in the freezer for up to 3 months. Defrost before using.

Another BOGOF recipe, the leftovers this time make pasties, which are perfect for the kids' tea the following day. Feel free to use diced lamb if you prefer. You can replace the pickled silverskin onions in the recipe with about 8–10 peeled shallots or pickling onions, halved if large, or 1 large onion, thickly sliced, along with 1 tablespoon balsamic vinegar.

Simple Beef and Barley Casserole

MAKES 2 adult and 4 kid-sized portions
PREPARATION TIME 20 minutes
COOKING TIME 2 hours

750g/1lb 10oz braising steak, cut into small cubes
2 tbsp plain/all-purpose flour
150g/5½oz pickled silverskin onions
2 celery stalks, cut into chunks
2 carrots, peeled and cut into chunks
375g/13oz butternut squash, peeled, deseeded and cut into chunks
75g/2½oz/⅓ cup pearl barley, rinsed well in cold water
2 tbsp demerara sugar
2 tsp Worcestershire sauce
2 tbsp tomato purée/paste
1 large thyme sprig and 2 bay leaves, tied with a piece of string
500ml/17fl oz/2 cups beef stock
250ml/9fl oz/1 cup red wine
sea salt and freshly ground black pepper
cabbage or curly kale, to serve (optional)

1 Preheat the oven to 160°C/315°F/gas 2–3.

2 Toss the beef in the flour and season well with salt and pepper. This can either be done in a bowl or a large freezer bag. Put the meat in a large flameproof casserole dish with all the remaining ingredients. Stir to mix everything together, then bring to the boil over a high heat. Cover with a lid and bake for 2 hours.

3 Serve the casserole just as it is or with some lovely buttery cabbage or curly kale.

Leftovers for lunchbox pasties
beef and barley pasties
Take a sheet of **ready-rolled puff** or **shortcrust pastry** and cut out circles, as big or small as you like or depending on how much of the casserole you have. Brush the edges with **beaten egg** and spoon some **cold casserole** in the middle, making sure you don't use much of the sauce. Fold up the edges of the pastry and pinch to seal. Pierce a hole in the pastry to allow any steam to escape when cooking. Brush with egg, put on a greased baking sheet and cook in a preheated oven at 200°C/400°F/gas 6 for 20–25 minutes until golden.

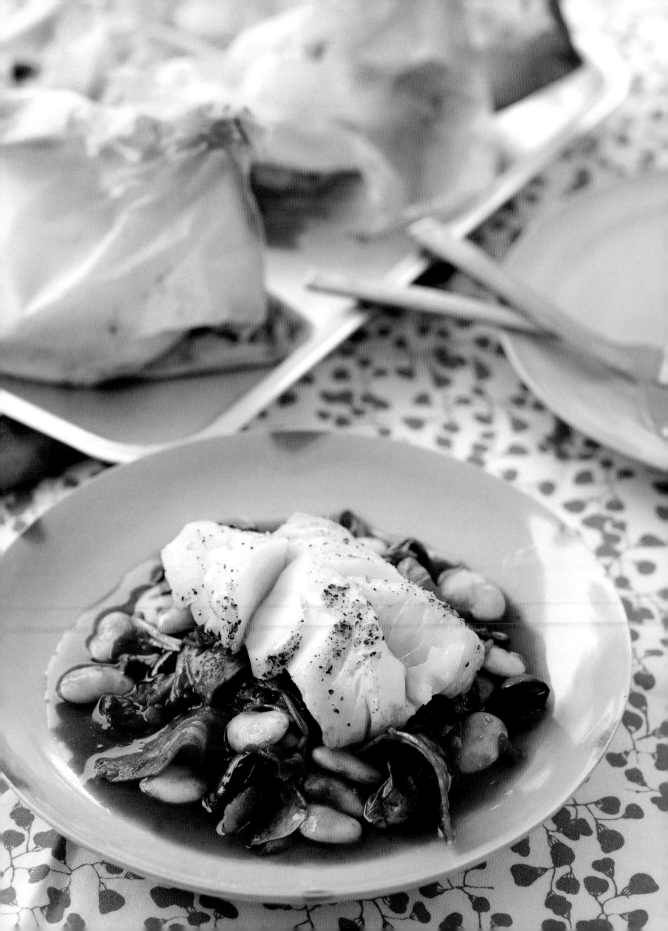

If you like the idea of very little washing up when you finally get the kids to bed so you can enjoy a meal with your partner, you're going to love this. It's a complete meal cooked all together in the oven (on a baking sheet) in a baking paper bag. The best thing to do is to prepare ahead (perhaps when the kids are eating their tea) and keep it in the refrigerator to cook later on in the evening.

Baked Fish in a Bag with Tomatoes, Butter Beans and Chorizo

MAKES 2 adult or 4 kid-sized portions
PREPARATION TIME 10 minutes
COOKING TIME 20 minutes

400g/14oz/1¾ cups canned chopped tomatoes
240g/8½oz canned butter beans, drained
90g/3¼oz/⅔ cup pitted black olives
1 bottled or canned roasted red pepper, sliced
10–12 thin slices of chorizo (about 40g/1½oz), halved
2 large handfuls of baby or young spinach leaves
2 fish fillets, such as cod, pollack, haddock or salmon
extra virgin olive oil, for drizzling
sea salt and freshly ground black pepper

1 Preheat the oven to 220°C/425°F/gas 7 and put a large baking pan in the oven to heat.

2 Take a piece of baking paper about 60–80cm/24–32in long and fold in half to make it double thickness, then fold in half again. Tightly fold together to seal two of the edges, creating a pouch, making sure there are no gaps for the food to escape when cooking. Repeat with another piece of baking paper. (Alternatively, you can buy baking paper bags from supermarkets that are all ready to use.)

3 Divide the tomatoes between the parcels, then do the same with the butter beans, olives, red pepper, chorizo and spinach. Season inside the bags with salt and pepper, then put the cod on top of the spinach. Season the fish and finish with a drizzle of extra virgin olive oil. Seal the open end of the bags by folding the edges over, leaving as much space in the bags as possible for steam to circulate when cooking. (The parcels can be prepared in advance and kept in the refrigerator for a good few hours before cooking.)

4 Put the parcels in the hot baking pan and bake for 20 minutes until the fish is cooked through. When cooked, split open the parcels and serve hot.

Make this recipe when you have a spare hour or so to leave it bubbling away, and serve it as a big family sit-down-together dish (it would stretch to a few stray kids too). It could be frozen as individual portions to get out as and when you need them or as something to give your kids for tea (as can many recipes in this chapter) and something for the grown-ups later in the evening. It's the recipe that keeps on giving. Keep it simple and serve with rice and add some extras, such as grated cheese, sour cream, shop-bought or Home-made Guacamole (see page 18) and wedges of lime.

Vegetable and Beany Gonzales Chilli

MAKES 6 adult and 6 kid-sized portions
PREPARATION TIME 15 minutes
COOKING TIME 1 hour

2 tbsp olive oil
1 large onion, chopped
2 peppers, red, green, yellow or orange, deseeded and diced
2 garlic cloves, crushed
2 courgettes/zucchini, diced
800g/1lb 12oz/3½ cups canned chopped tomatoes
480g/1lb 1oz canned red kidney beans, drained
2 tsp ground cumin
1½ tsp mild chilli powder (or hot if you want added heat)
1 tsp ground cinnamon
2 tsp unsweetened cocoa powder
1 tbsp chopped coriander/cilantro leaves (optional)
sea salt and freshly ground black pepper
cooked long-grain rice, to serve

1 Heat the oil in a large pan over a low heat, add the onion and peppers and cook for 5 minutes until beginning to soften. Add the garlic and courgettes/zucchini and cook for a further 3–4 minutes.

2 Stir in all the remaining ingredients along with 125ml/4fl oz/½ cup water and season lightly with salt and pepper. Increase the heat and bring to the boil, then reduce the heat, cover loosely with a lid and leave to simmer for 45 minutes, stirring a couple of times.

3 Scatter with the coriander/cilantro leaves, if using, and serve with rice.

Leftovers for Tex-Mex tacos
chilli tacos and chilli baked wedges

If you want to serve this chilli in a different way – perhaps for a lighter meal – then pop **1 handful of shredded crispy lettuce**, such as iceberg, into a **taco shell**. Add a large **spoonful of the chilli** and top with **grated cheese**. Serve with **sour cream** and/or **guacamole**, **lime wedges** and **Tabasco sauce** for added heat, if you fancy it.

Or you could cook wedges of **potato** or **sweet potato** following the recipe on page 148, or use shop-bought ones, if preferred. When cooked, transfer to individual ovenproof dishes, or one large one if you are going to share, and spoon over some of the **leftover chilli**. Scatter with **plenty of grated Cheddar cheese** and pop in a preheated oven at 200°C/400°F/gas 6 for about 15 minutes until the chilli is heated through and bubbling hot.

This Moroccan-inspired dish ticks so many boxes. It's healthy, comforting, full of flavour, quick and can easily be increased to serve more people – although these portions are fairly generous. What's more, the kids love the sweetness coming from the sweet potatoes and dried apricots. If you have extra sweet potatoes, they are great baked in a hot oven for about 45 minutes, then served with a knob of butter and lots of freshly ground black pepper.

Chickpea and Sweet Potato Get-you-out-of-a Stew

MAKES 2 adult and 4 kid-sized portions
PREPARATION TIME 10 minutes
COOKING TIME 1 hour

4 tbsp olive oil
2 red or white onions, thickly sliced
6 garlic cloves, crushed
2 tsp ground cinnamon
2 tsp turmeric
2 tsp ground cumin
2 tsp paprika
1 tsp ground ginger
¼ tsp cayenne pepper
800g/1lb 12oz/3½ cups canned chopped tomatoes
480g/1lb 1oz drained canned chickpeas/garbanzos
4 carrots, peeled and cut into large chunks
4 sweet potatoes, peeled and cut into large chunks
200g/7oz/1 heaped cup dried, ready-to-eat apricots, torn in half
2 large handfuls of coriander/cilantro leaves, chopped
juice of 2 lemons

1 Heat the oil in a large flameproof casserole, or a tagine if you have one. Add the onions and cook over a low heat with the lid on for about 10 minutes until softened and starting to colour, stirring a couple of times during cooking. Stir in the garlic and spices and cook for a minute or so before adding 400ml/14fl oz/scant 1¾ cups water and all the remaining ingredients except the chopped coriander/cilantro and lemon juice.

2 Bring to a simmer and cover loosely with a lid. Leave to simmer for up to 45 minutes until the sweet potatoes and carrots are tender.

3 Add the coriander/cilantro and lemon juice, stir through and serve.

This is a good standby meal in our house, as I always have peas and broad/fava beans in the freezer, risotto rice in the cupboard and a few additional bits in the refrigerator. If you want to be a bit more fancy, you can also use fresh peas, broad/fava beans and other veggies, such as green beans or asparagus. They'll just need cooking for a few minutes in boiling water before you add to the risotto. And if you've ever wondered what to do with leftover risotto, here's your answer. It's worth making this recipe just to try out my Mozzarella and Primavera Arancini Cakes.

Baked Risotto Primavera

MAKES 2 adult and 4 kid-sized portions
PREPARATION TIME 10 minutes
COOKING TIME 25 minutes

2 tbsp olive oil
1 tbsp butter
1 large onion, chopped
3 garlic cloves, crushed
2 courgettes/zucchini, diced
275g/9¾oz/1¼ cups carnaroli or arborio risotto rice
1l/35fl oz/4 cups hot chicken or vegetable stock
grated zest of 1 small lemon
125g/4½oz/scant 1 cup frozen peas, defrosted
125g/4½oz/scant 1 cup frozen broad/ fava beans or soy beans, defrosted
3 tbsp chopped chives, mint, basil or parsley leaves (or a mixture)
50g/1¾oz/⅔ cup cup freshly grated Parmesan cheese
3 tbsp mascarpone or cream cheese
sea salt and freshly ground black pepper

1 Preheat the oven to 200°C/400°F/gas 6.

2 Heat the oil and butter in a small flameproof casserole dish over a low heat, add the onion and garlic and fry for 5 minutes until softened. Add the courgettes/zucchini and rice and stir around until coated in the oil.

3 Stir in the stock and bring just to the boil, then cover with a lid and bake for 15 minutes. If you are around, give it a stir halfway, but it's not essential. By now the rice will be just tender and most of the liquid absorbed. Stir in the peas and broad/fava beans and return to the oven for 5 minutes.

4 Finally, when the risotto is ready, stir in the chopped herbs, lemon zest, Parmesan and mascarpone. Season lightly with salt and pepper and serve hot.

Leftovers Italian style

mozzarella and primavera arancini cakes
For every **200g/7oz/1¼ cups leftover risotto**, mix in **25g/1oz diced mozzarella** and **3 finely chopped sun-dried tomatoes**. Firmly shape into 2 cakes. Dip into some **beaten egg** and then into **3–4 tbsp fresh or dried breadcrumbs**. Heat enough **olive oil** in a frying pan to cover the base of the pan, add the arancini and fry over a medium heat for 3–4 minutes on each side until golden and heated through. Drain on paper towels and serve.

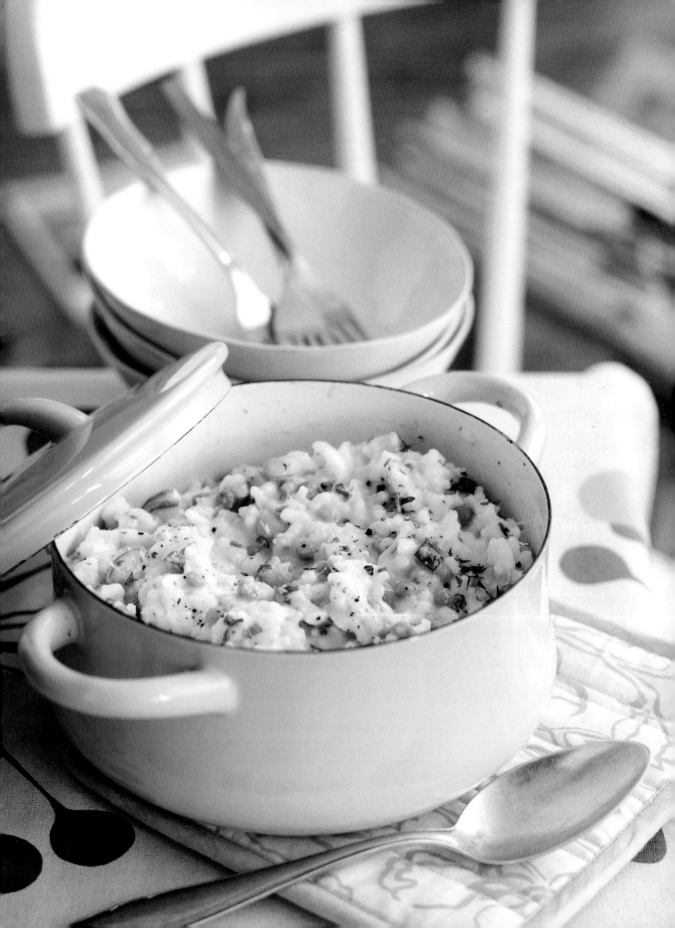

These can be made and eaten straight away or popped in the refrigerator and enjoyed within a couple of days. My mum used to make a similar dessert to this and hide a surprise in the bottom – chocolate buttons, pieces of fruit or little sweets. I now realize that she successfully used this as a way of encouraging me to eat up. Clever Mum!

Fruity Fools with a Hidden Surprise

MAKES 2 adult or 4 kid-sized portions
PREPARATION TIME 10 minutes for soft fruits or 15 minutes, plus cooling, for hard fruits

80ml/2½fl oz/⅓ cup double/heavy or whipping cream
80ml/2½fl oz/1⅓ cup shop-bought or Foolproof Home-made Custard (see page 128) or Greek yogurt
125ml/4½fl oz/½ cup fruit purée (see method) or shop-bought fruit compôtes or pie fillings

FOR THE FRUIT PURÉE
250g/9oz/1⅔ cups hard fruits, such as chopped rhubarb or peeled, cored and chopped apples or pears
or 250g/9oz/1⅔ cups fresh or frozen soft fruits, such as berries, frozen smoothie mixes, pitted and peeled mango or pitted cherries, defrosted if frozen
sugar, to taste

FOR THE SURPRISE
a few chocolate buttons, candy sweets or pieces of fresh or dried fruit (optional)

1 To make a fruit purée, prepare your chosen fruit as necessary. If you are using hard fruits, they will need cooking. Put them in a pan over a medium heat with 2 tbsp water, bring to the boil, then reduce the heat to medium-low, cover with a lid and leave to simmer until the fruit has softened. Add sugar to taste and briskly stir or whizz in a blender until smooth. Leave to cool. If using soft fruits, put the fruit into a blender and whizz until smooth. Taste and add sugar if needed.

2 To make the fools, whisk the cream until it forms soft peaks. Fold in the custard and the fruit purée, either until totally combined or creating a marbled effect.

3 Put a little surprise at the bottom of individual glasses or bowls, if you like, and spoon in the fool over the top. Either chill in the refrigerator or eat straight away.

leftovers for iced treats
frozen fools and fool ice cream
Rather than eating straight away as a dessert, the fool mixture can be transformed into two very handy treats.

To make Frozen Fools, spoon the **fool** into moulds and pop in the freezer. The lollies/popsicles will last for a couple of months and are great for emergencies or hot sunny days.

If you have an ice cream machine, the **fool** mix can be churned to create a lovely, creamy, fruity Fool Ice Cream. Store in an old ice cream container or a plastic box with a lid and it will be waiting for you in the freezer to tuck into and enjoy whenever the sun shines.

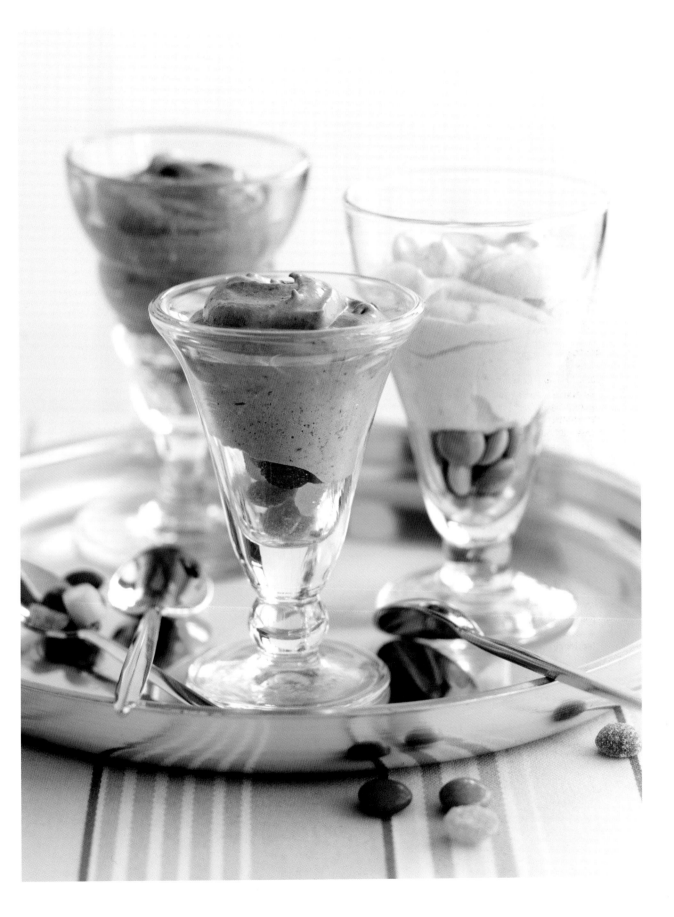

If there is ever a time when you want to say 'well done' – whether it is for a good mark at school, doing well at sports, tidying up a bedroom or just for good behaviour – an indulgent sundae is the best way to say it (well, it works in my house).

Well Done Mondaes to Fridaes

MAKES about 250ml/9fl oz/1 cup sauce
PREPARATION TIME 5 minutes
COOKING TIME 5 minutes

FOR THE HOT CHOCOLATE FUDGE SAUCE
100g/3½oz dark chocolate, 70% cocoa
  solids, broken into small pieces
2 tbsp unsweetened cocoa powder
115g/4oz golden/light corn syrup
80ml/2½fl oz/⅓ cup double/heavy
  cream
40g/1½oz/⅓ cup icing/confectioners'
  sugar
½ tsp vanilla extract
a pinch of salt

FOR THE SUNDAE
ice cream
decorations, such as:
• crumbled meringues or biscuits/cookies
• sliced bananas or other favourite fruit
• whipped cream (this is a bit over the
  top but if they deserve it, then so be it!)
• popping candy/space dust
• over-the-top decorations, such as
  wafers, paper umbrella, sparklers,
  morello cherries

1 To make the fudge sauce, put the chocolate and unsweetened cocoa powder in a large heatproof bowl. Rest the bowl over a pan of gently simmering water, so that the bottom of the bowl does not touch the water. Stir occasionally until the chocolate has melted. (Alternatively, you can do this in the microwave in 5-second bursts on Defrost or Low.) Remove from the heat and stir in all the remaining ingredients until smooth and well blended.

2 Layer up the sundae ingredients in tall sundae glasses or ice cream bowls and add whatever decorations you like. Spoon a little of the sauce over the ice cream and serve straight away.

Lifesaver topping
hot chocolate fudge sauce

Once you have spooned some sauce over the ice cream, leave the rest to cool, then transfer to a glass jar with a lid and store in the refrigerator for up to 4 weeks. You can serve it cold or gently heat whatever quantity you need.

Having a jar of home-made chocolate fudge sauce in your refrigerator is dangerous, of course, as it's very tempting to dip your finger into it every time you see it! But it will be a real hit spooned over an **ice cream sundae**, as a **pancake filling, poured over chocolate cake or pudding** or spread **on top of cupcakes**.

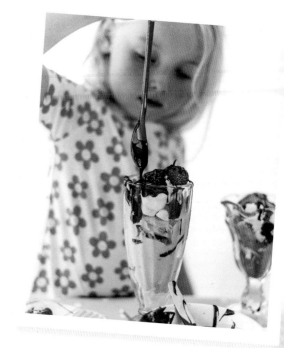

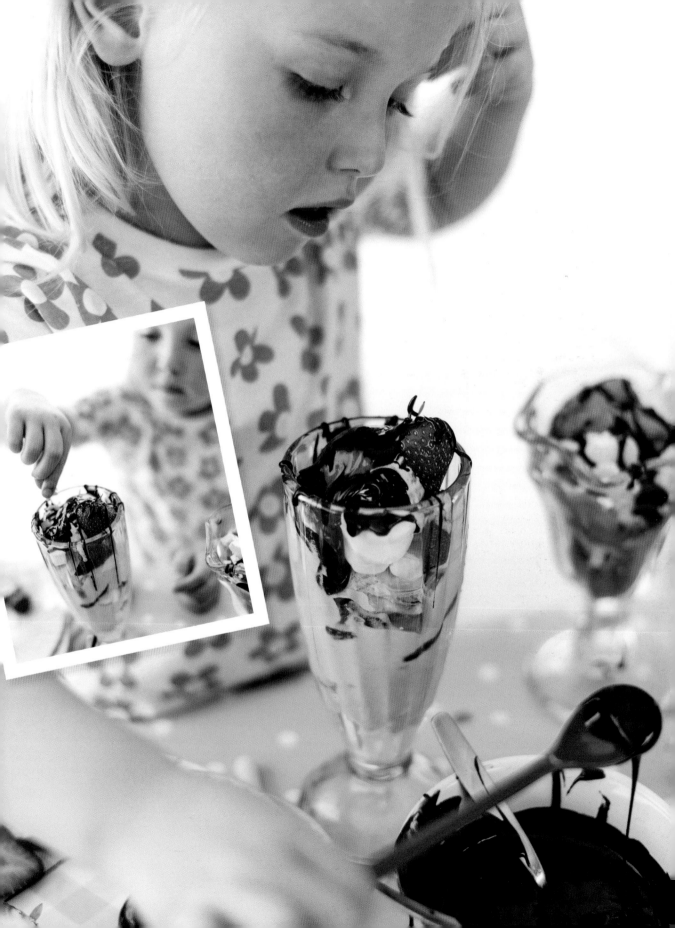

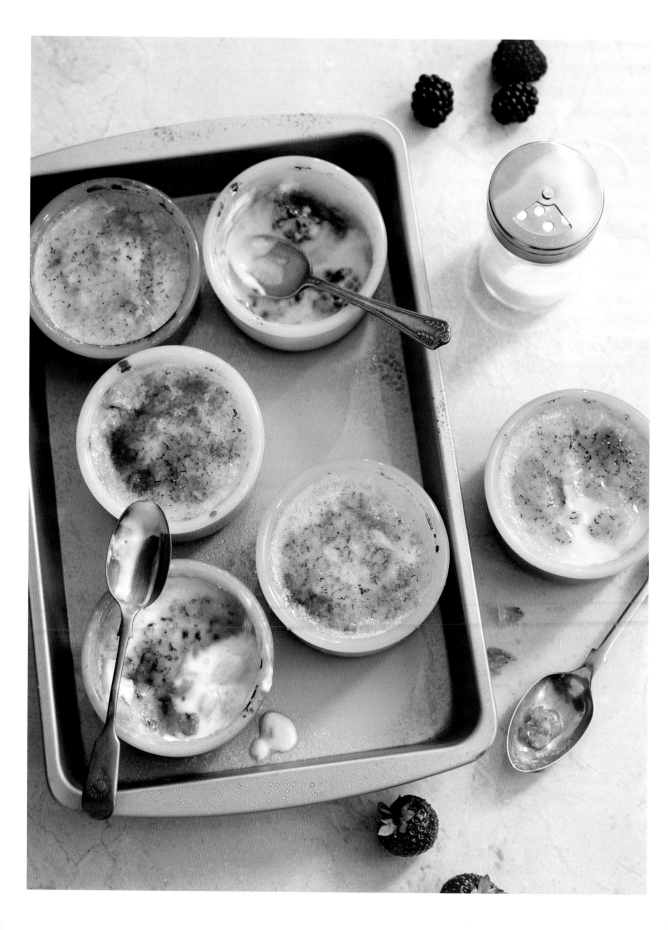

A midweek restaurant-style pudding that will certainly beat having plain fruit or yogurt for dessert any day of the week. Of course, if you have a kitchen blowtorch, using that will be quicker than putting it under the grill/broiler, and adds drama to the recipe. The best bit of all is cracking the top of the brûlées with the spoon – the kids love it (and so do I!).

Fruit and Yogurt Brûlées

MAKES 2 adult or 4 kid-sized portions
PREPARATION TIME 5 minutes
COOKING TIME 2 minutes

100–150g/3½–5½oz fresh soft fruit, such as plums, berries, banana or mango
a few drops of vanilla extract, rosewater or orange flower water
300ml/10½fl oz/scant 1¼ cups Greek yogurt
50g/1¾oz/scant ¼ cup caster/superfine sugar

1 If the fruit is large, cut it into smaller pieces and spoon into the base of individual ramekin dishes. Mix the vanilla extract into the yogurt and spoon on top of the fruit. Smooth over the surface, cover and keep in the refrigerator if not eating straight away.

2 Preheat the grill/broiler to its hottest setting. Sprinkle the caster/superfine sugar over the yogurt in a thick, even layer. Put the ramekins onto a baking sheet and grill/broil for 1–2 minutes until the sugar melts and is golden and bubbling. Remove from the grill/broiler and the sugar will set almost straight away. Serve immediately.

How to make
super caramel
If you think your grill/broiler just isn't quite powerful enough to make a decent caramel topping for the Fruit and Yogurt Brûlées, then fear not, it's very easy to make caramel separately in a pan. When you are ready to finish the crème brûlées, put the **50g/1¾oz/scant ¼ cup caster/superfine sugar** in a small saucepan over a low heat until it turns a deep caramel colour. Don't stir the sugar when it is caramelizing, but you can swirl the pan to ensure even colouring. Pour or spoon a little of the caramel over each crème brûlée, and leave for about a minute or so for the caramel to set before serving.

Crumbles make lovely comfort food with custard, cream or ice cream. For the filling, anything goes, but I've suggested some of those we like best and created different crumble toppings. Keep some of your favourite crumble mix in the freezer so you can simply make up your chosen filling and sprinkle it over the top.

Mix-and-Match Fruit Crumbles

MAKES 2 adult or 4 kid-sized portions, plus 10 adult portions
of the crumble mixes for the freezer
PREPARATION TIME 10 minutes, using a pre-made crumble mix or 15
minutes from scratch
COOKING TIME 20 minutes, or 30 minutes for apple and pear

SWEET CRUMBLE MIX

250g/9oz butter, diced
310g/11oz/scant 2½ cups plain/all-
   purpose flour
250g/9oz/1⅓ cups soft brown sugar
85g/3oz/scant 1 cup rolled oats
a large pinch of salt
2 tsp ground cinnamon, ground ginger
   or mixed spice (optional)
125g/4½oz/1 cup flaked/slivered
   almonds, lightly crushed

1 Lightly rub together the butter and flour until the mixture resembles coarse, slightly chunky breadcrumbs. Stir in the sugar, oats, salt, spice, if using, and almonds.

2 Reserve about 150g/5½oz/1½ cups for each two-person crumble. (Put the remainder in freezer bags in suitable quantities, label and freeze.)

GINGERNUT CRUMBLE MIX

150g/5½oz gingernut biscuits/cookies
250g/9oz butter, diced
310g/11oz/2½ cups plain/all-purpose
   flour
250g/9oz/scant 1¼ cups caster/
   superfine sugar
50g/1¾oz/½ cup rolled oats
a large pinch of salt
2 tsp ground ginger

1 Put the gingernuts in a sandwich bag and crush with a rolling pin until you have large crumbs. Lightly rub together the butter and flour until the mixture resembles coarse, slightly chunky breadcrumbs. Stir in the sugar, oats, crushed gingernuts, salt and spice.

2 Reserve about 150g/5½oz/1½ cups for each two-person crumble. (Put the remainder in freezer bags in suitable quantities, label and freeze.)

APPLE AND PEAR CRUMBLE

1 tbsp butter
2 apples, peeled, cored and diced
2 pears, peeled, cored and diced
1 tbsp caster/superfine sugar
150g/5½oz/1½ cups crumble mix
shop-bought or Foolproof Home-made
  Custard (see page 128), cream or ice
  cream, to serve

1 Preheat the oven to 200°C/400°F/gas 6.

2 Melt the butter in a saucepan with the fruit, sugar and 1 tbsp water. Cover and cook for 5 minutes, or until softened slightly. Spoon the filling into ovenproof dishes. Sprinkle your chosen crumble mix over the filling.

3 Bake for about 20 minutes until bubbling and golden. Serve with custard, cream or ice cream.

CHERRY AND CHOCOLATE CRUMBLE

375g/13oz canned pitted cherries,
  drained and juice reserved
75g/2½oz dark chocolate, 70% cocoa
  solids, or milk chocolate, broken into
  small pieces
150g/5½oz/1½ cups crumble mix
shop-bought or Foolproof Home-made
  Custard (see page 128), cream or ice
  cream, to serve

1 Preheat the oven to 200°C/400°F/gas 6.

2 Divide the cherries between two small ovenproof dishes. Spoon over enough syrup or juice to half cover them. Sprinkle with the chocolate, then with your chosen crumble mix.

3 Bake for about 20 minutes until bubbling and golden. Serve with custard, cream or ice cream.

FROZEN BERRY AND ORANGE CRUMBLE

grated zest of ½ orange
2 tbsp caster/superfine sugar
300g/10½oz frozen mixed berries,
  defrosted
150g/5½oz/1½ cups crumble mix
shop-bought or Foolproof Home-made
  Custard (see page 128), cream or ice
  cream, to serve

1 Preheat the oven to 200°C/400°F/gas 6.

2 Stir the orange zest and sugar into the fruit. Spoon into ovenproof dishes. Sprinkle your chosen crumble mix over the filling.

3 Bake for about 20 minutes until bubbling and golden. Serve with custard, cream or ice cream.

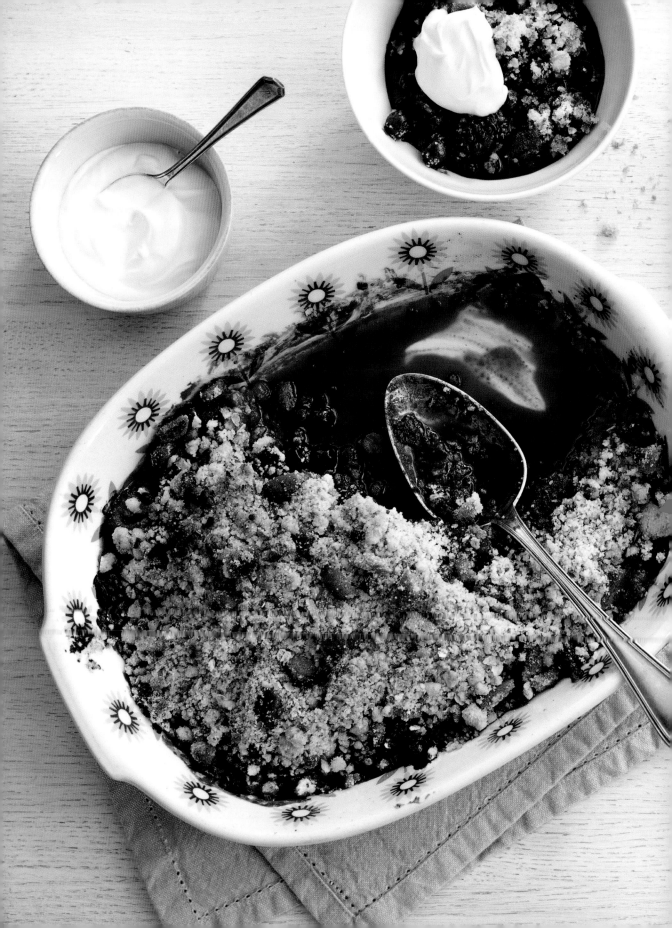

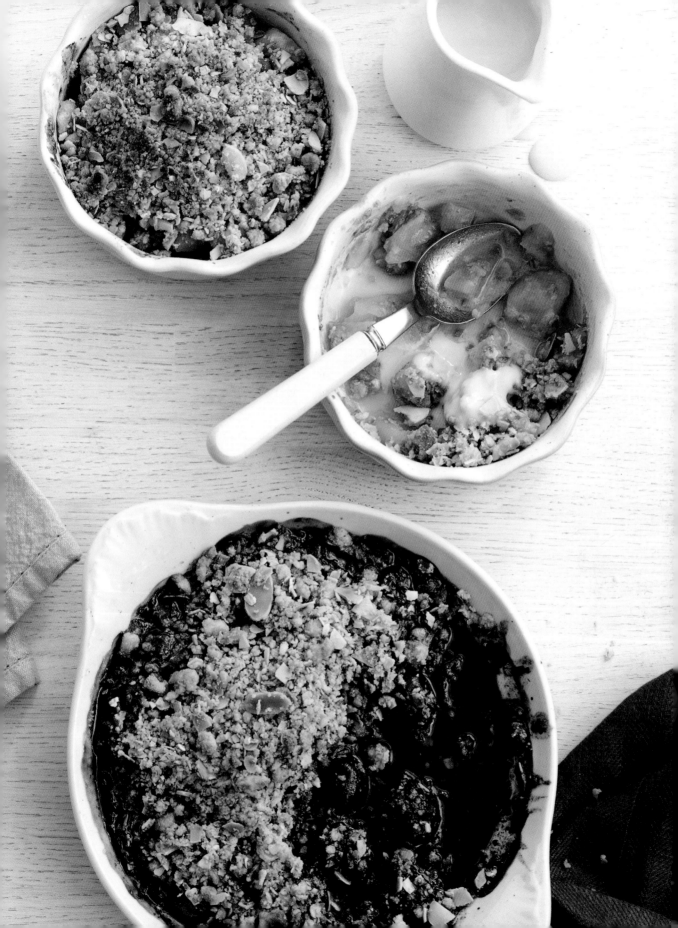

This is a great excuse to use up any leftover cooked rice. If you don't have any, it'll just take a little longer to make (or you could buy a packet of pre-cooked rice). It works with other fruits, too, instead of bananas. Try raspberries, strawberries, mango or pear. If you have no fruit, it still tastes delicious just as a simple chocolate rice pudding.

Chocolate and Banana Rice Pudding

MAKES 2 adult or 4 kid-sized portions
PREPARATION TIME 5 minutes
COOKING TIME 20 minutes

200g/7oz/1¼ cups cooked or leftover basmati or long-grain rice
500ml/17fl oz/2 cups milk, plus extra if required
50g/1¾oz dark chocolate, 70% cocoa solids, broken into pieces
50g/1¾oz/scant ¼ cup caster/superfine sugar
2 bananas, peeled and sliced

1 Put the rice and milk in a non-stick saucepan. Bring to the boil over a high heat, then reduce the heat to low and leave to simmer gently for 20 minutes until thickened, stirring occasionally.

2 Add the chocolate and sugar and stir gently until melted. Remove the pan from the heat and stir in extra milk, if necessary, if the mixture appears too thick.

3 Either stir the bananas into the chocolate rice pudding, then spoon into a bowl, or arrange the bananas on top. Serve your rice pudding hot. (If you have any left over, chill and eat cold within a day.)

Leftovers for a treat
melting marshmallow arancini

This is a little treat the kids will love – so much so that you might want to make extra of the pudding just so you get one as well. Using wet hands to stop the mixture sticking to you, roll the **leftover pudding** into little balls about the size of a golf ball. Push your finger into the centre, push a **mini marshmallow** into the hole, then close the rice over the hole. Roll the balls in **beaten egg**, then in some **crushed biscuits** or **cookies**. Heat a little **butter** or **butter and oil** in a frying pan, add the arancini and fry gently until golden and fragrant, turning them frequently. Serve hot, warm or cold.

I have to admit, when chocolate is a must, these extremely quick and easy puddings are my guilty little pleasure. They are designed specifically for the microwave and are a true lifesaver. Stick to the basic pudding or, for an additional treat, add a little surprise to them from the suggestions below. The cooking times are based on an 850-watt microwave. It's pretty amazing to see these puddings cook in a matter of minutes.

Lifesaver Speedy Chocolate Puddings

MAKES 2 adult or 4 kid-sized portions
PREPARATION TIME 5 minutes
COOKING TIME 2 minutes

FOR THE CHOCOLATE PUDDINGS
3 tbsp sunflower, vegetable, rapeseed/
   canola or groundnut oil, plus extra
   for greasing
4 tbsp self-raising flour
4 tbsp caster/superfine sugar
3 tbsp unsweetened cocoa powder
3 tbsp milk
1 egg
½ tsp vanilla extract

SUGGESTIONS FOR THE EXTRA TREATS
choose your favourites, such as:
• 1–2 tbsp chocolate chips or drops
• a scattering of mini marshmallows
• 2 tsp jam
• finely grated orange zest
• 1 tbsp chopped roasted hazelnuts
   or other nuts
• ½ banana, peeled and chopped

ice cream, cream or crème fraîche,
   to serve (optional)

1 Greased two microwave-safe teacups, small mugs or ramekin dishes with oil. Mix together all the pudding ingredients until you have a smooth batter and divide evenly between the prepared dishes. If you are adding an extra treat, gently stir it in.

2 Put in the microwave and cook on High for 2 minutes.

3 Tuck in either as they are, or turn out into bowls and enjoy with a spoon of ice cream, cream or crème fraîche, if you like.

Lifesaver dessert
speedy lemon syrup puddings
If it isn't chocolate you are craving but just something comforting in a matter of minutes, you can easily take the basic recipe and tweak it around a little to suit you. The unsweetened cocoa powder can be replaced with **extra flour** and you can add additional flavours as you like, such as **grated orange zest**, **ground ginger**, **ground cinnamon**, **almond extract** and so on. Here's how to make a lemon syrup pudding. Mix together **6 tbsp self-raising flour** with **1 tbsp caster/superfine sugar, 2 tbsp golden/light corn syrup, 3 tbsp oil, 3 tbsp milk, 1 egg** and the **finely grated zest of ½ lemon**. Cook as above.

Every household that includes kids has to contain jam tarts. These are simple to make and a lovely recipe to bake with the children. In the unlikely event that you don't eat all the jam tarts within a couple of days, don't let them go to waste – simply warm them through in the oven and serve with custard or transform into Jammy Apple Bakewells (see below).

Jammy Apple Tarts

MAKES 12 tarts
PREPARATION TIME 5 minutes
COOKING TIME 15 minutes

melted butter, for greasing
about 325g/11½oz ready-rolled shortcrust pastry
12 tsp jam, whichever flavour you like
1 apple, peeled, cored and thinly sliced
2 tbsp desiccated/dried shredded coconut or crushed flaked/slivered almonds
icing/confectioners' sugar, for dusting (optional)
shop-bought or Foolproof Home-made Custard (see page 128) (optional), to serve

1 Preheat the oven to 200°C/400°F/gas 6. Use a pastry brush to brush the holes of a shallow patty or bun pan with a little melted butter.

2 Using a cutter, cut out 12 circles of pastry to fit the holes of the pan and lightly press into the holes. Put 1 tsp jam in each one, then lay the sliced apple on top. Scatter over the coconut or almonds and dust each one with icing/confectioners' sugar, if you like.

3 Bake for 12–15 minutes until the pastry is golden, the jam is bubbling and the apple is becoming golden.

4 While hot, carefully transfer to a wire rack and leave to cool. Serve warm or cold, dusted with more icing/confectioners' sugar, and with custard, if you like.

Leftovers for almond cakes
jammy apple bakewells

If you don't manage to finish up all the tarts, you can use them as a base for some mini bakewells. Line a muffin pan with paper cases – about twice as many as you have leftover tarts. Roughly cut the **leftover tarts** into 1cm/½in pieces and divide evenly between the cases. Beat together **100g/3½oz softened butter** with **115g/4oz/½ cup caster/superfine sugar**, then gradually add **3 beaten eggs** alternately with **150g/5½oz/1½ cups ground almonds** and **1 tsp almond extract**. This quantity will make 6 generous muffins so adjust the quantities accordingly. Spoon the bakewell mixture into the muffin cases and bake in a preheated oven at 190°C/375°F/gas 5 for about 25 minutes until risen and golden. Serve hot or cold.

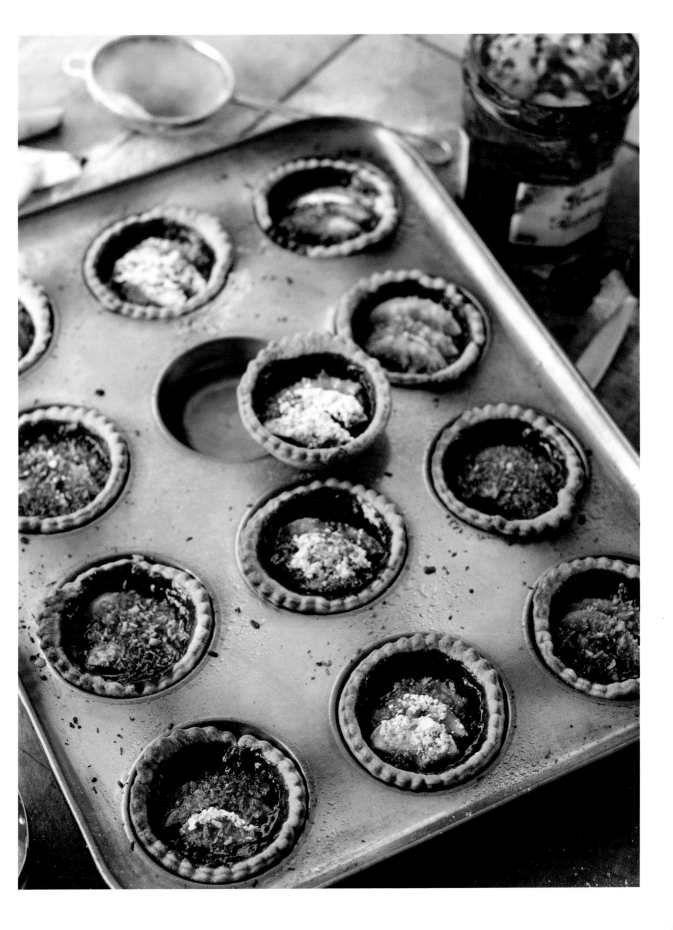

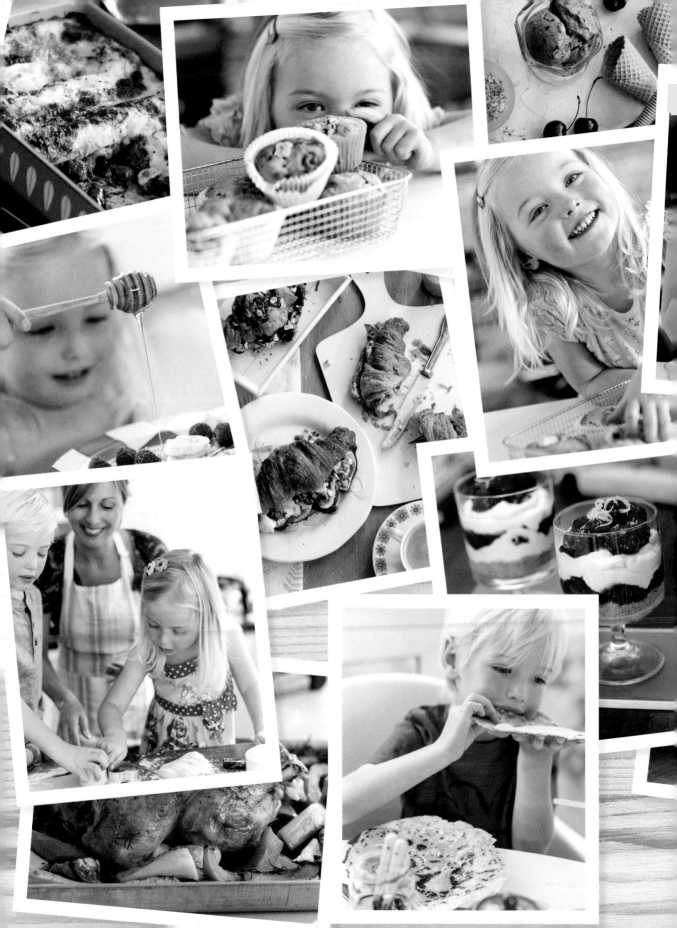

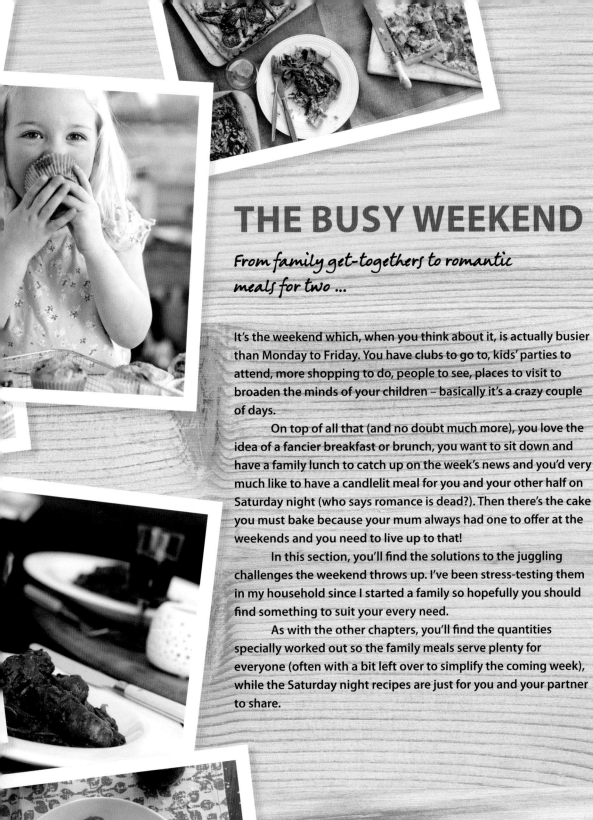

THE BUSY WEEKEND

From family get-togethers to romantic meals for two ...

It's the weekend which, when you think about it, is actually busier than Monday to Friday. You have clubs to go to, kids' parties to attend, more shopping to do, people to see, places to visit to broaden the minds of your children – basically it's a crazy couple of days.

On top of all that (and no doubt much more), you love the idea of a fancier breakfast or brunch, you want to sit down and have a family lunch to catch up on the week's news and you'd very much like to have a candlelit meal for you and your other half on Saturday night (who says romance is dead?). Then there's the cake you must bake because your mum always had one to offer at the weekends and you need to live up to that!

In this section, you'll find the solutions to the juggling challenges the weekend throws up. I've been stress-testing them in my household since I started a family so hopefully you should find something to suit your every need.

As with the other chapters, you'll find the quantities specially worked out so the family meals serve plenty for everyone (often with a bit left over to simplify the coming week), while the Saturday night recipes are just for you and your partner to share.

Even if your kids are not big on eating fruit or drinking milk on its own, they should enjoy drinking one of these fruity options. In fact, most adults I know love them too. Decorate with extra fruit, maple syrup or honey, if you like.

Milkshakes

EACH ONE MAKES 2 large or 4 small shakes
PREPARATION TIME 3 minutes

STRAWBERRY OR RASPBERRY SHAKE

400ml/14fl oz/scant 1¾ cups milk
200g/7oz/1⅓ cups strawberries or
    raspberries, stalks removed
½ tsp vanilla extract
4–6 ice cubes
clear honey or maple syrup, to taste
    (optional)

1 Pour the milk into a blender. Add the fruit, vanilla extract and ice cubes and whizz for 30–45 seconds until smooth. Add honey or maple syrup to taste, if you like.

2 Strain into glasses to remove any pips or chunks of ice and serve.

BANANA AND PEANUT BUTTER SHAKE

400ml/14fl oz/scant 1¾ cups milk
2 ripe bananas, peeled and roughly
    chopped
2 tbsp peanut butter
4–6 ice cubes
clear honey, to taste

1 Pour the milk into a blender. Add the bananas, peanut butter and ice cubes and whizz for 30 seconds until smooth. Add a little honey to taste.

2 Strain into glasses to remove chunks of ice and serve.

VANILLA AND MAPLE SYRUP SHAKE

400ml/14fl oz/scant 1¾ cups milk
2 tbsp maple syrup
1 tsp vanilla extract
4–6 ice cubes

1 Pour the milk into a blender. Add the maple syrup, vanilla extract and ice cubes and whizz for about 15 seconds until smooth.

2 Strain into glasses to remove chunks of ice and serve.

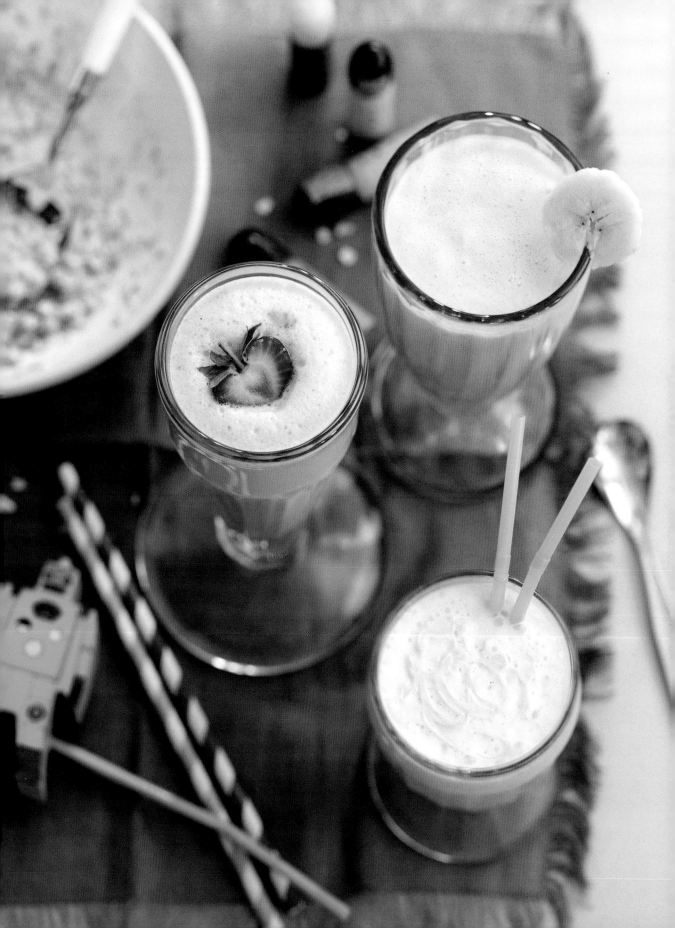

If you're feeling a little rough around the edges from clinging on to your social life the night before and need some help in getting through the morning, a classic Bloody Mary should do the trick. If you still feel rough later on, use what tomato juice you have left and make a chilled Gazpacho Soup (see below).

Classic Bloody Mary

MAKES 2 glasses
PREPARATION TIME 5 minutes

100ml/3½fl oz/scant ½ cup vodka
300ml/10½fl oz/scant 1¼ cups tomato
  juice
a good squeeze of lemon juice
6–8 drops of Worcestershire sauce
3–4 drops of Tabasco sauce
a pinch of celery salt (optional)
freshly ground black pepper
ice

1 Measure the vodka and tomato juice into tall glasses.

2 Add the remaining ingredients to taste, stir together – and enjoy.

Leftovers for summer soup
gazpacho soup

If you have opened up a carton or bottle of tomato juice, you can use any left over in all types of recipes. Use it as an alternative to milk in savoury scones, instead of water in bread, in pasta sauces, casseroles and hot soups. Plus you can turn it into a delicious chilled soup that is a summery favourite. Blend together **2 ripe tomatoes, ¼ onion, ¼ cucumber, ½ red pepper, 1 garlic clove, 1 tbsp extra virgin olive oil, 1 tsp sherry** or **white wine vinegar, a dash of Tabasco** and **350ml/12fl oz/scant 1½ cups tomato juice** and season to taste with **sea salt** and **freshly ground black pepper** to give you a thick soup consistency. Serve chilled. This makes enough for 2 adult portions.

This is so easy to do – and if you have leftover cooked sausages, it's quick too. If you don't – or you don't have time to cook them – just make ordinary eggy bread instead.

Sausage Eggy Bread

MAKES 2 adult and 2 kid-sized portions
PREPARATION TIME 5 minutes
COOKING TIME 15 minutes

sunflower oil, for frying
6 pork sausages, split in half lengthways
4 eggs
6 tbsp milk
6 slices of fresh white bread
tomato ketchup, brown sauce, mustard,
   sweet chilli sauce or barbecue sauce
50g/1¾oz butter
sea salt and freshly ground black pepper

1 Heat a little oil in a large frying pan over a medium heat, add the sausages and fry for about 5 minutes until golden and cooked through.

2 Meanwhile, beat together the eggs and milk in a wide, shallow bowl and season lightly with salt and pepper.

3 When the sausages are cooked, lay them onto 3 slices of bread. Spread over some of your chosen sauce, then top with the other slices of bread. Press down firmly to seal. Lay the sandwiches in the egg mixture and leave to soak for about 2 minutes. Carefully turn them over and soak for a further 2–3 minutes until the egg mixture has been absorbed.

4 Wipe out the pan with paper towels and put over a medium heat. Add the butter and, once it is bubbling, put the sandwiches in the pan. (If your pan isn't big enough to fit the sandwiches, use just half the butter and cook one at a time.) Cook for 3–4 minutes on each side until puffed up and golden, turning carefully with a spatula.

5 When cooked, halve one of the sandwiches for the kids and serve with extra sauce of your choice.

According to my kids, this is what Woody and Jessie from *Toy Story* eat for breakfast every day to make them so strong. You can actually serve this dish any time of the day – I quite like it on a baked potato when I'm in on my own, or back home late and want something quick and hearty.

Cowboy Beans-on-toast

MAKES 2 adult and 2 kid-sized portions
PREPARATION TIME 2 minutes
COOKING TIME 10 minutes

a drizzle of olive oil
4 pork sausages, skinned
820g/1lb 13oz/3¼ cups canned baked beans
barbecue sauce or smoked paprika, to taste
a couple of drops of Tabasco sauce (optional)
brown or white bread, toasted and buttered

1 Heat a frying pan or saucepan over a medium-high heat and add the oil, then break the sausages into the pan in chunks. Fry for 5 minutes until the sausages are golden and cooked through, breaking down any larger chunks of the sausages with a wooden spoon.

2 Add the baked beans and bring to the boil, then reduce the heat, stir in some barbecue sauce to taste and cook for a few minutes to thicken. Add the Tabasco sauce if you fancy a spicy kick.

3 Spoon onto buttered toast and off you go … Yeehaa!

Leftovers for sausage pies
cowboy pasties
Take a sheet of **ready-rolled puff** or **shortcrust pastry** and cut out circles, as big or small as you like, or depending on how much of the cowboy beans you have left over. Brush the edges with **beaten egg** and spoon the cold filling in the middle. Add some **grated cheese** if you fancy it, too. Fold up the edges of the pastry and pinch together to seal. Pierce a hole in the pastry to let any steam escape when cooking. Brush with **egg**, put on a greased baking sheet and bake in a preheated oven at 200°C/400°F/gas 6 for 20–25 minutes until golden.

Easy to prepare and delicious served with a toasted muffin, this is really a dish for you and your partner, so you can add a splash of Tabasco for a kick if you like. If you are using ham, it doesn't matter what type – Parma ham is particularly delicious. If you want to make this into more of a light lunch recipe, the addition of some wilted spinach or a few fried sliced mushrooms – or both – at the bottom of the dishes makes it extra special. And, of course, you can easily increase the quantities to serve more people.

Baked Eggs with Smoked Salmon or Ham

MAKES 2 adult portions
PREPARATION TIME 5 minutes
COOKING TIME 12 minutes

about 1 tbsp butter, for greasing
2–4 slices of smoked salmon or ham
2 eggs
2 tbsp cream
2 tsp chopped chives (optional)
1 tbsp finely grated Parmesan cheese
sea salt and freshly ground black pepper
toasted and buttered English muffins or toast, to serve

1 Preheat the oven to 220°C/425°F/gas 7 and grease two individual ovenproof dishes, such as ramekins, with butter. If you don't have any dishes, a deep muffin pan will do.

2 Put the smoked salmon or ham into the dishes, pushing it down into the edges to create a bowl shape. Break an egg into each one, then pour over the cream. Season lightly with salt and pepper, scatter over the chives, if using, and finish with the cheese.

3 Bake for 12 minutes until the egg white is only just set and the yolk is still runny. The eggs will continue to cook once removed from the oven so don't be tempted to leave them in the oven too long if you still want a runny yolk.

4 Serve either in the baking dishes or turned out, with toasted buttered muffins or toast.

Forget heading for the same butter and jam on your weekend croissant – these are much more exciting combinations. The quantities listed for each one will fill two croissants.

Baked Croissants

EACH ONE MAKES 2 croissants
PREPARATION TIME 5 minutes
COOKING TIME 5 minutes

FIG, GOATS' CHEESE AND WALNUT CROISSANTS

2 croissants, split open
2 ripe figs, sliced
50g/1¾oz crumbly goats' cheese
1 small handful of walnut pieces
clear honey, to taste

1 Preheat the oven to 200°C/400°F/gas 6.

2 Put the bottom half of the croissants on a baking sheet. Put the figs on top, then scatter over the cheese and walnuts. Replace the tops. Bake for 4–5 minutes until heated through. Drizzle with honey to taste. Leave the croissants for a minute or so to cool slightly, then serve.

RICOTTA, PARMA HAM, AVOCADO AND CHILLI CROISSANTS

2 croissants, split open
4 tbsp ricotta cheese
2–4 slices of Parma ham
1 ripe avocado, pitted, peeled and sliced
a pinch of dried chilli/hot pepper flakes
sea salt and freshly ground black pepper

1 Preheat the oven to 200°C/400°F/gas 6.

2 Put the bottom half of the croissants on a baking sheet. Spread with the ricotta and top with the Parma ham, sliced avocado and chilli/hot pepper flakes. Season lightly with salt and pepper. Replace the tops. Bake for 4–5 minutes until heated through. Leave to cool slightly, then serve.

CHOCOLATE, BANANA AND ALMOND CROISSANTS

2 croissants, split open
100g/3½oz dark chocolate, 70% cocoa
  solids, or milk chocolate, broken into
  small pieces
1 small banana, peeled and sliced
1 small handful of toasted flaked/
  slivered almonds
icing/confectioners' sugar, for dusting

1 Preheat the oven to 200°C/400°F/gas 6.

2 Put the bottom half of the croissants on a baking sheet. Scatter most of the chocolate over the top, plus all the banana and almonds, then replace the tops. Finely chop the remaining chocolate and scatter over the croissants. Bake for 4–5 minutes until they are crisp outside and oozing chocolate. Dust with icing/confectioners' sugar, leave to cool slightly, then serve.

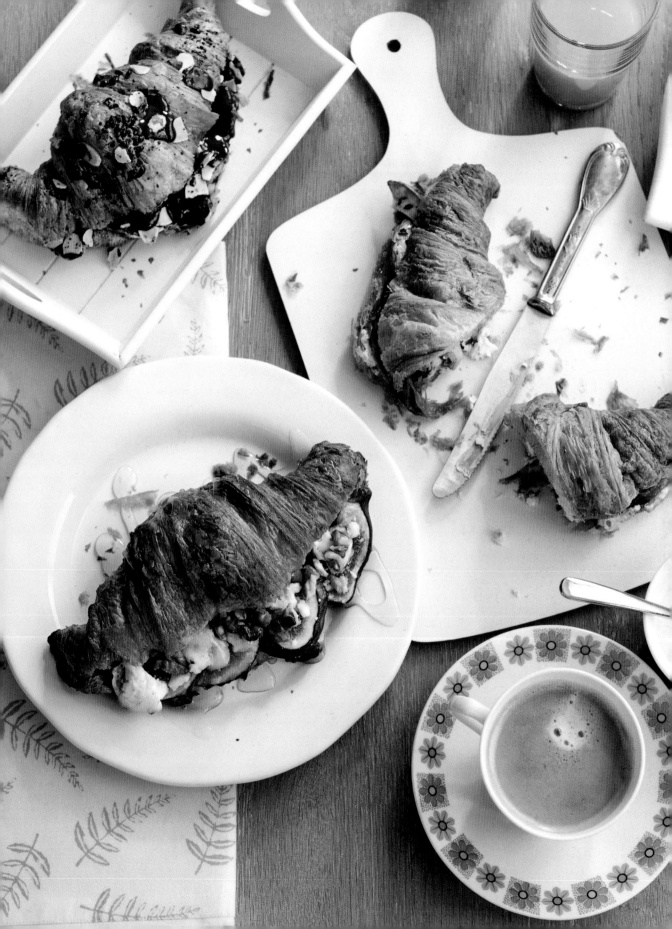

Can you ever remember the quantities when you are making pancakes? How often do you end up calling your mum? Well it's worth investing in some measuring cups or finding a teacup that is 250ml/9fl oz – this makes it so much easier to memorize the quantities (just don't forget which mug or tea cup you used). American-style pancakes tend to be thicker and smaller. If you want French crêpes, use a large pan and add the minimum amount of batter to thinly cover the base of the pan.

Foolproof Pancakes

MAKES 12–14 American-style or 8–10 crêpes
PREPARATION TIME 5 minutes
COOKING TIME 4 minutes each

125g/4½oz/1 cup self-raising flour (either plain/all-purpose or self-raising can be used for crêpes)
250ml/9fl oz/1 cup milk (just under for American-style, just over for crêpes)
1 egg
a pinch of salt
butter or sunflower oil, for frying

SUGGESTIONS TO SERVE
try some of these options:
• clear honey, golden/light corn syrup, maple syrup or jam
• Hot Chocolate Fudge Sauce (see page 64), chocolate spread or caramel sauce
• fresh fruit, such as berries or bananas
• grated lemon or orange zest and sugar
• yogurt
• ice cream … for breakfast? I know some of you will!

1 Put the flour, milk, egg and salt in a blender or food processor and mix together well. Alternatively, use a bowl and whisk until smooth. The consistency should be that of double/heavy cream for crêpes, so add a little extra milk if you need to. (Cook straight away or chill for up to 24 hours until needed – loosen with extra milk if necessary.)

2 Heat a pancake or frying pan over a medium-high heat and add a small piece of butter or a trickle of oil until it melts all over the base of the pan. Add a spoonful of the batter, rolling the pan to spread it over the base of the pan, and cook for a couple of minutes on each side until golden. Keep the pancakes warm while you cook the remaining pancakes.

3 Serve with your chosen topping and enjoy.

Leftovers for Sunday roast
yorkshire puddings
Any pancake batter that hasn't been used up is brilliant for making Yorkshire puddings. Keep the batter covered in the refrigerator. When you are ready to cook, put a good drizzle of sunflower oil in each hollow of a shallow bun or patty pan and put the pan in the oven while it heats to 220°C/425°F/gas 7. After 5 minutes, quickly take out the pan and pour the **batter** into the holes, filling them halfway. Return to the oven on the top shelf and cook for 12–15 minutes until golden and risen. Serve with your roast dinner or as a snack topped with **baked beans** and **cheese**, or even as a dessert drizzled with **clear honey, golden/light corn syrup** or **maple syrup** and **lemon juice**.

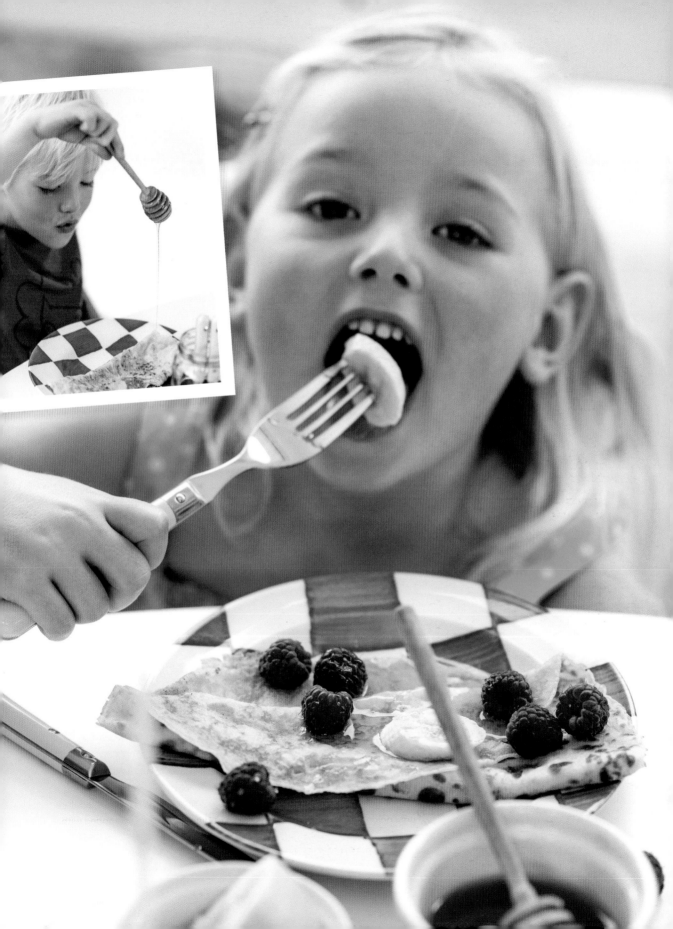

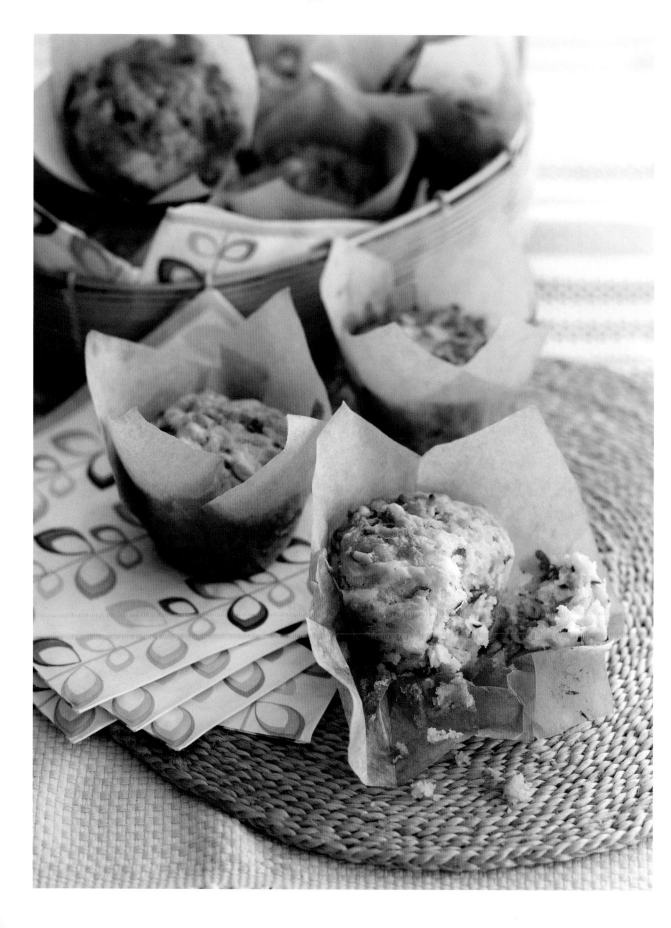

We all need snack ideas to avoid resorting to the cookie pan, and this recipe is one to add to your armoury. They are light and extremely tasty and perfect for eating when you are on the go.

Savoury Muffins

MAKES 12 muffins
PREPARATION TIME 15 minutes
COOKING TIME 20 minutes

butter, for greasing (optional)
40g/1½oz/scant ⅓ cup pine nuts
225g/8oz/scant 2 cups self-raising flour
2 tsp baking powder
100g/3½oz/⅔ cup polenta or semolina
150g/5½oz/1¼ cups grated mature
  Cheddar cheese
150g/5½oz courgettes/zucchini, grated
2 eggs
200ml/7fl oz/scant 1 cup plain yogurt
80ml/2½fl oz/⅓ cup olive or rapeseed/
  canola oil
75g/2½oz ham, salami or chorizo, finely
  chopped
sea salt and freshly ground black pepper

1 Preheat the oven to 180°C/350°F/gas 4 and line a 12-hole muffin pan with paper muffin cases. Alternatively, lightly grease the holes of the muffin pan, then press a 13cm/5in square of baking paper into each hole, shaping the squares to fit by folding the sides.

2 Put the pine nuts in a dry, non-stick pan over a medium heat for a few minutes, shaking and tossing the pan continuously until they start to turn golden. (Don't leave them in the pan or they will quickly burn.) Tip them out onto a plate to cool.

3 Mix together the flour, baking powder and polenta in a mixing bowl.

4 In a separate bowl, lightly mix together two-thirds of the cheese and all the remaining ingredients. Pour the wet ingredients into the dry ingredients and mix quickly and lightly to form a lumpy batter. (Over-mixing will make the cooked muffins turn out heavy.) Spoon into the prepared muffin cases and scatter the remaining cheese over the top. Bake for 20 minutes until risen and golden.

5 Leave to cool in the pan for a few minutes, then transfer to a wire rack. Serve warm or cold.

Leftovers are lovely toasted
toasted muffins
The muffins are lovely as a picnic lunch served with some tomato chutney, or for a weekday packed lunch. After a day or so, they will become a little dry, but are delicious split in half and lightly toasted under the grill/broiler, spread with **butter** or **cream cheese** and topped with **chutney** or **tomato salsa**.

This recipe is hearty and flavoursome in the tradition of the Italian classic, the name of which means 'big soup' – it's also quick and easy to make. You don't have to be strict about the ingredients you use – it really is a case of whatever veg you can find in the drawer in the refrigerator and any shape pasta you happen to have. Any leftovers can be heated up the next day with an extra splash of water if it's too thick (and a cheeky splash of dry sherry when serving, if it's a tough day!).

Easy Minestrone Soup

MAKES 2 adult and 2 kid-sized portions
PREPARATION TIME 10 minutes
COOKING TIME 20 minutes

2 tbsp olive oil
1 onion, chopped
2–4 smoked streaky bacon rashers/
   slices, diced (optional)
2 garlic cloves, crushed
2 celery stalks, finely sliced
3 veggies from your refrigerator, about
   200g/7oz, chopped, such as courgette/
   zucchini, carrot, small red pepper,
   handful of green beans, small leek
750ml/26fl oz/3 cups hot vegetable
   stock
750g/1lb 10oz/3 cups canned chopped
   tomatoes or passata/Italian sieved
   tomatoes
75g/2½oz spaghetti or linguine, broken
   into small pieces, or small pasta shapes
sea salt and freshly ground black pepper

TO SERVE
green pesto (optional)
freshly grated Parmesan cheese

1 Heat the oil in a saucepan over a medium heat, add the onion and bacon, if using, and cook for 5 minutes until the onion is beginning to soften. Stir in the garlic, celery and any chopped vegetables and cook for about 5 minutes.

2 Add the stock, tomatoes and pasta, bring to the boil, then reduce the heat to medium and leave to simmer for 10 minutes, or until the vegetables and pasta are all tender. Season lightly with salt and pepper.

3 Ladle the soup into bowls, top with a spoonful of pesto, if you like, and serve sprinkled with grated Parmesan.

How to make

parmesan croûtons

If you have a loaf of bread that's gone beyond its best, don't just give it all to the ducks. Have a go at making some cheese croûtons to scatter over your weekend soup. To make enough for 4 adult-sized portions, simply remove the crusts from **2–3 slices of bread** and cut each piece into about 1cm/½in cubes. Toss with **2 tbsp olive oil** and **2 tbsp finely grated Parmesan cheese**. Tip onto a baking sheet and bake in a preheated oven at 220°C/425°F/gas 7 for 10–12 minutes until golden and crunchy, turning a couple of times. Leave to cool slightly.

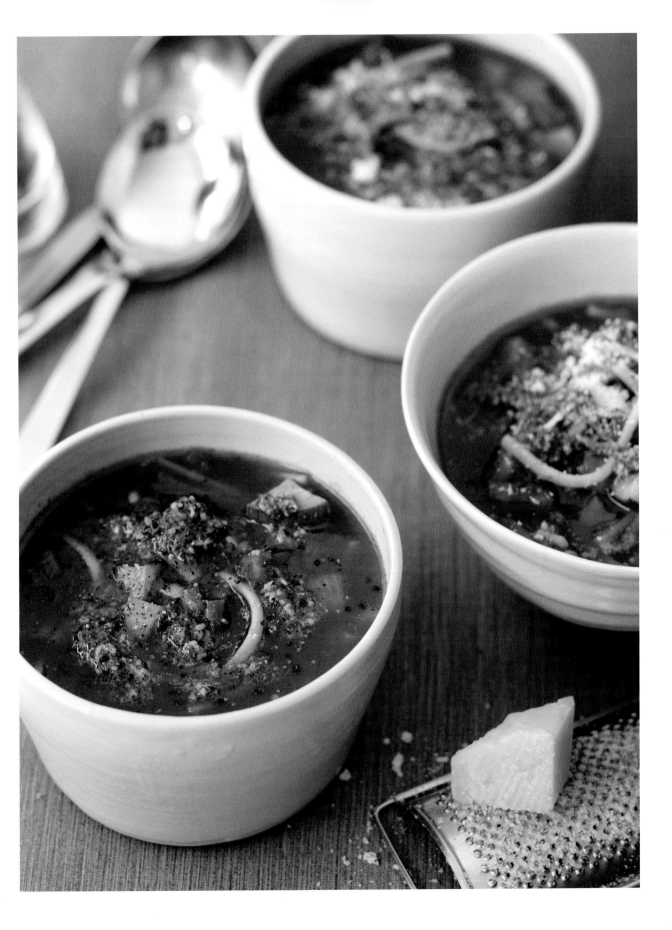

Part-baked baguettes are a really convenient standby to have in your cupboard for those occasions when you've eaten all the bread at breakfast and haven't made it to the shops yet. You can adapt the recipe to use whatever different flavour combinations you like, such as mozzarella, roasted red pepper, pesto and Parma ham, or Stilton, spinach leaves, avocado, tomato chutney or even caramelized onions.

Baked Baguettes with your Favourite Fillings

MAKES 2 baguettes
PREPARATION TIME 10 minutes
COOKING TIME 15 minutes

2 part-baked baguettes, white or brown
175g/6oz/scant 1½ cups grated mature Cheddar cheese
2–4 slices of ham, torn into pieces (optional)
2–4 spring onions/scallions, finely chopped
2–3 tbsp mayonnaise
3 sun-dried tomatoes, chopped
1 small handful of basil leaves, torn into pieces
sea salt and freshly ground black pepper (optional)

1 Preheat the oven to 200°C/400°F/gas 6.

2 Split the baguettes in half lengthways and put the base of each one on a large piece of foil. Mix together the cheese, ham, if using, spring onions/scallions and mayonnaise. Season lightly with salt and pepper, if you like. Spread the mixture over the bottom halves of the baguettes, top with the sun-dried tomato and basil and put the other half of the bread on top. Fold the foil up the sides of the bread to cover it loosely, leaving the top open.

3 Bake for 12–15 minutes, turning over halfway through. Remove from the foil and leave to cool slightly, then serve.

Kids love burgers and if you make your own, you know that they are made with healthy ingredients. You can easily double the quantities to make more – so they are perfect for when your children invite their friends round for lunch or tea.

Burger in a Bun with Cheese

MAKES 4 large or 6 small burgers
PREPARATION TIME 25 minutes
COOKING TIME 8 minutes

FOR THE BURGERS
500g/1lb 2oz minced/ground beef
1 small onion, finely chopped
2 garlic cloves, crushed
2 tsp Dijon mustard
1 tbsp Worcestershire sauce
1 egg yolk
oil, for brushing
sea salt and freshly ground black pepper
1 recipe quantity Perfect Coleslaw (see below), to serve

TO SERVE
burger buns or ciabatta rolls, split in half
¼ iceberg lettuce, shredded
3 tbsp mayonnaise
1–2 tomatoes, sliced
4–8 slices of melting cheese, such as mature Cheddar, Gruyère, Taleggio or blue cheese
1 red onion, sliced
gherkins/cornichons, sliced (optional)
tomato ketchup or mustard

1 Put all the burger ingredients except the oil in a bowl and mix well, preferably using your hands. Firmly shape into burgers. (Cook straight away or chill until needed.)

2 When you're ready to cook the burgers, heat a griddle or frying pan until it is really hot. Brush with a little oil and cook the burgers for about 8 minutes, turning them every minute or so. Alternatively, cook on a hot barbecue (the coals should be glowing white) for the same amount of time. Constantly turning them will keep them moist and allow them to cook evenly.

3 While the burgers are cooking, lightly toast the burger buns or ciabatta rolls. Mix the lettuce with the mayonnaise and divide evenly onto the bottom halves of the rolls, then top with the tomatoes. As soon as the burgers are cooked, top with the cheese so it instantly starts to melt. Put the burgers on top of the tomatoes, then finish with some red onion and gherkin/cornichon, if using, tomato ketchup or mustard. Serve with coleslaw.

How to make
perfect coleslaw

This has to be the perfect side dish to many meals, especially these burgers and the Speedy Steak and Pan-fried Avocado Club Sarnie (see page 24). Very **thinly slice ½ red** or **white cabbage** and **1 small red** or **white onion** using the fine slicer blade on a food processor, a mandolin or a sharp knife. Then **coarsely grate 2 carrots** and mix with the cabbage and onion. In a separate bowl, mix together **4 tbsp plain yogurt, 2 tbsp mayonnaise, 1½ tsp Dijon mustard, 1 tbsp olive oil** and **1 tbsp white wine vinegar**. Season with a little **sea salt** and **freshly ground black pepper**, then mix together the dressing and the vegetables. Keep in the refrigerator and use within a couple of days. This makes enough for 2 adult and 2 kid-sized portions.

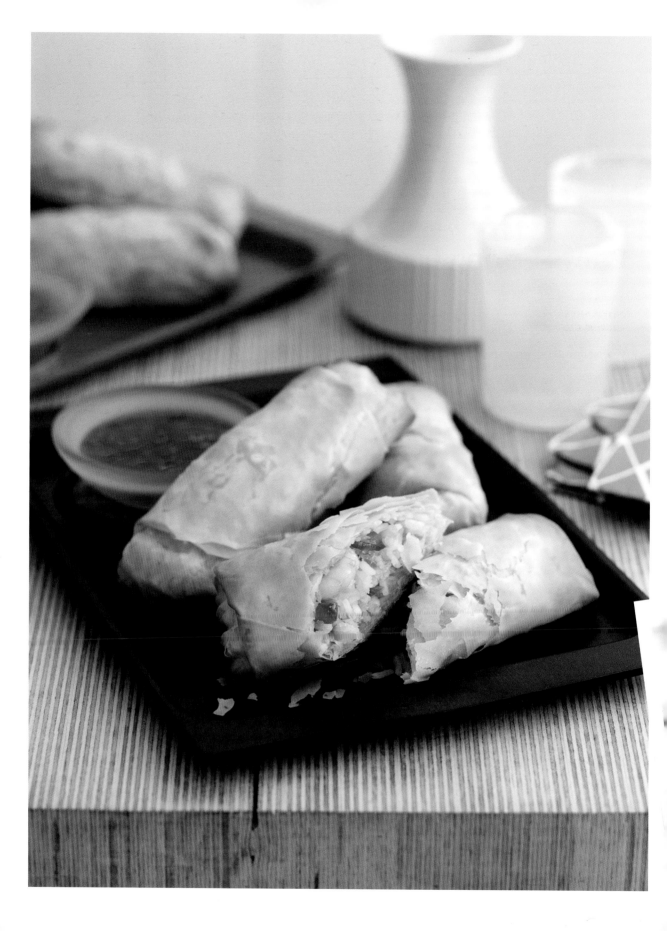

Get the kids involved in making these. They are fun and extremely tasty. Filo/phyllo pastry is a great standby and here wraps up a rice, prawn/ shrimp and vegetable filling, but you could use your imagination to add other ingredients, depending on what you have in the cupboard or the refrigerator. Flaked canned tuna works well, as does shredded cooked chicken or extra vegetables.

Prawn Spring Rolls

MAKES 6 rolls
PREPARATION TIME 15 minutes
COOKING TIME 18 minutes

FOR THE PRAWN/SHRIMP FILLING
250g/9oz/1⅓ cups cooked basmati rice (using shop-bought pre-cooked, leftovers or freshly cooked)
100g/3½oz cooked, peeled prawns/ shrimp
100g/3½oz carrots, peeled and grated
½ red pepper, deseeded and diced
1–1½ tsp sweet chilli dipping sauce, plus extra to serve (or tomato ketchup if preferred)

FOR WRAPPING
6 sheets of fresh filo/phyllo pastry, cut into 12 23cm/9in squares
sunflower or vegetable oil, for brushing

1 Preheat the oven to 220°C/425°F/gas 7.

2 Mix together all the filling ingredients in a bowl. Lay a sheet of filo/ phyllo pastry on the work top or board and brush lightly with oil. Put another sheet of pastry on top and brush lightly with oil. Turn the square so that one corner of the pastry is pointing towards you.

3 Spoon about one-sixth of the filling onto the corner nearest you. Fold this corner towards the centre and tuck it under the filling. Fold the two outside corners to the middle so it looks like an envelope. Brush lightly with oil, then roll up to look like a sausage shape. Brush once more and put it on a non-stick baking sheet. Repeat until you have made the rest of the spring rolls. (Cook straight away or chill until needed.)

4 Bake for 15–18 minutes until the rolls are lightly golden and crisp. Leave to cool slightly, then serve with extra sweet chilli dipping sauce or tomato ketchup.

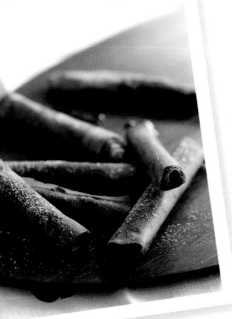

Leftovers with filo and chocolate sweet sticks

If you had to cut rectangles of filo/phyllo pastry into squares and you've ended up with some **pastry trimmings**, they can be used to make chocolate or jam sweet sticks. Carefully spread **1–2 tsp chocolate and hazelnut spread** or **jam** in a fairly even layer on top of the pastry, then roll up down the length of the pastry, creating a stick shape. Brush with a little **oil** and dust with **icing/confectioners' sugar**. Put on a non-stick baking sheet and bake in a preheated oven at 220°C/425°F fan/gas 7 for about 8 minutes until golden.

Quick and easy, this uses ingredients you should be able to get from the local shop and makes the perfect light snack for your weekend. If you don't have canned potatoes, you can boil up your own potatoes and cut into cubes, then follow the recipe.

Cornershop Pepper and Feta Frittata

MAKES 2 adult and 2 kid-sized portions
PREPARATION TIME 10 minutes
COOKING TIME 20 minutes

2 tbsp olive oil
1 red or white onion, chopped
2 garlic cloves, crushed
500g/1lb 2oz canned new potatoes, drained and cut into cubes
2 bottled or canned roasted red peppers, cut into strips
155g/5½oz/1 cup frozen peas, defrosted
1 small handful of parsley leaves, chopped
6 eggs, beaten
200g/7oz feta cheese, crumbled
sea salt and freshly ground black pepper
mixed salad, to serve

1 Heat the oil in a flameproof 20cm/8in non-stick frying pan over a medium heat, add the onion and cook for about 5 minutes until softened and just beginning to turn golden. Add the garlic and cubed potatoes and continue to cook for about 3 minutes until the potatoes are thoroughly heated through.

2 Stir the red peppers, peas and parsley into the beaten eggs, season lightly with salt and pepper, then pour the mixture into the pan and scatter the feta cheese over the top. Reduce the heat to as low as possible and cook the frittata for about 10–12 minutes until it is almost set – carefully checking the underneath isn't burning by lifting the edge of the frittata with a spatula.

3 Meanwhile, preheat the grill/broiler to high. Put the pan under the grill/broiler for a couple of minutes to cook the top of the frittata and give it a slightly golden appearance.

4 Slide onto a plate, cut into wedges and serve with salad.

Leftovers for pasta
red pepper pesto

Use up any roasted peppers to make a delicious pesto sauce. Lightly toast **50g/1¾oz/⅓ cup pine nuts** in a dry frying pan until just becoming golden. Tip into a food processor and add **1 crushed garlic clove**, **1 large handful of basil leaves**, **50g/1¾oz/⅔ cup freshly grated Parmesan cheese**, **125ml/ 4fl oz/½ cup olive oil** and **1 roasted red pepper**. Season lightly with **sea salt** and **freshly ground black pepper** and blitz until smooth. Use straight away or pour into a clean jar, cover with a little extra oil, seal with a lid and store in the refrigerator for up to a week.

Aarrrrgh! It's lunchtime, you're all hungry and your plan was to go shopping after lunch to stock up, so there's nothing in the house. Well, have a dig around in the refrigerator for an onion, grab a potato and some veg out of the freezer and you're almost good to go.

Frozen Vegetable Soup

MAKES 2 adult and 2 kid-sized portions
PREPARATION TIME 10 minutes
COOKING TIME 15 minutes

25g/1oz butter
1 small onion, chopped
2 garlic cloves, crushed
1 small potato, peeled and diced
1 bay leaf (optional)
500ml/17fl oz/2 cups hot vegetable
 or chicken stock
350g/12oz frozen vegetables (peas,
 carrots, sweetcorn – whatever you
 have)
2 tbsp mascarpone, cream cheese or
 cream
sea salt and freshly ground black pepper
crusty bread, to serve

FOR THE FLAVOURINGS
if you are using a single vegetable, it is nice to add some extra flavours, for example:
• cauliflower: add 1 tsp Dijon mustard to the soup and stir through some grated Cheddar at the end rather than the mascarpone or cream cheese
• peas: sauté a few bacon rashers/ slices with the onion, and add 2 tbsp chopped mint leaves at the end
• broccoli: add a good grating of nutmeg, and stir in an extra 2 tbsp cream cheese at the end, or the addition of some blue cheese is particularly nice if you have any

1 Heat the butter in a large saucepan over a medium heat and when it is bubbling, add the onion, garlic, potato and bay leaf, if you have one. Cover with a lid and cook over a medium heat for 10 minutes, stirring a couple of times.

2 Add the stock and bring to the boil. Stir in the vegetables, return to the boil and cook for 5 minutes until the vegetables are tender. Remove the bay leaf, if you were using one, and blitz the soup with a hand blender or in a blender until it is smooth.

3 For a creamy finish, stir in the mascarpone and season lightly with salt and pepper. Stir in any extra flavourings, if you like.

4 Serve hot with crusty bread to dip in.

Leftovers for another day
garlic croûtons
There are no rules for making this kind of soup, just use whatever you have to hand, things you want to use up, or random items from the veggie rack. Just don't use too many strongly flavoured vegetables – taste as you go along. It's quite likely you'll end up with more than you need for one sitting, but you'll certainly not waste it. Serve it for lunch the next day, perhaps sprinkled with some **freshly grated Parmesan cheese** or some **garlic croûtons**, made by quickly frying **cubes of bread** in **hot oil** with a **crushed garlic clove**. Or simply allow the soup to cool, pack in plastic boxes in suitable quantities, label and put in the freezer so it is there to save the day another time.

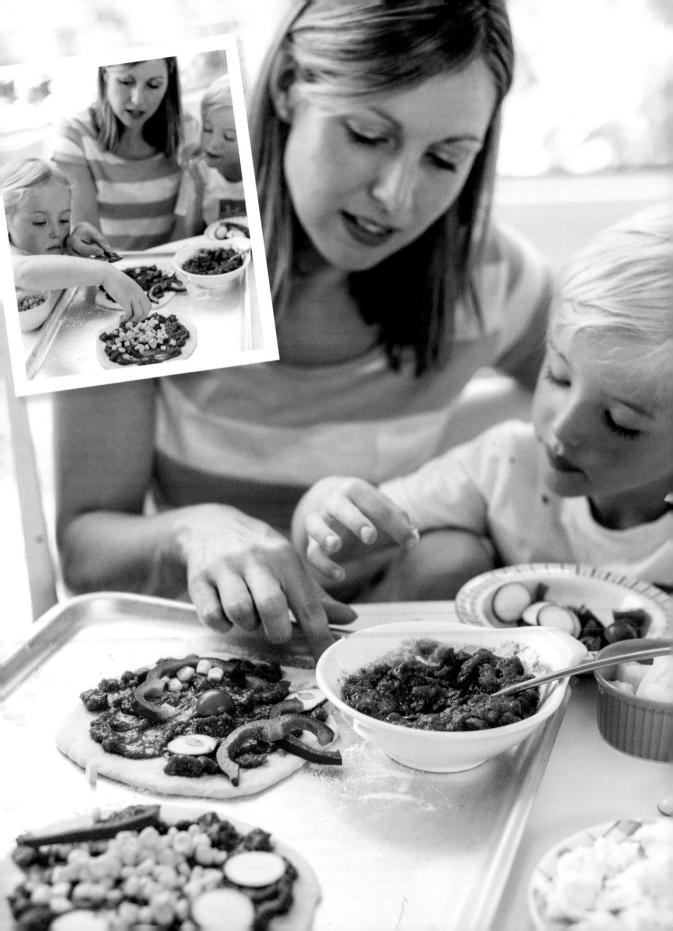

Making pizzas with the kids is great fun. This is a basic Margherita, but you can add any topping you like. My favourite is nuggets of sausage meat, broccoli florets and dried chilli/hot pepper flakes, but ricotta cheese, Parma ham, sun-blush tomatoes and olives comes a close second. The kids love making faces with chunks of vegetables.

Pizza Art

MAKES 2 large or 4 small pizzas
PREPARATION TIME 20 minutes, plus
  30 minutes rising (optional)
COOKING TIME 10 minutes

FOR THE PIZZA DOUGH
300g/10½oz/scant 2½ cups strong
  white bread flour, plus a little extra
  for dusting
1 tsp instant yeast
1 tsp salt
1 tbsp olive oil

FOR THE TOMATO AND MOZZARELLA
  TOPPING
150ml/5fl oz/scant ⅔ cup Tomato Sauce
  (see below) or passata/Italian sieved
  tomatoes
1 handful of basil leaves, torn or roughly
  chopped
250–350g/9–12oz mozzarella, torn into
  pieces
olive oil, for drizzling
plus any of your favourite toppings
  as extras

1 Put the flour, yeast and salt in bowl and make a well in the centre. Pour in the oil and 200ml/7fl oz/scant 1 cup lukewarm water and bring the ingredients together with a wooden spoon or your hands until you have a soft, fairly wet dough. Turn out onto the surface dusted with flour and knead for a good 5 minutes until smooth and elastic. Alternatively you can mix everything together in a food mixer with a dough hook.

2 If you have the time, put the dough in a clean, lightly oiled bowl and cover with a piece of oiled cling film/plastic wrap. Leave in a warm place for about 30 minutes. It's not essential to do this for a thin crust pizza but it will make a lighter dough.

3 Preheat the oven to 240°C/475°F/gas 8. Put two baking sheets in the oven on separate shelves to preheat and lightly flour two baking sheets.

4 Knead the dough quickly if you left it to rise, then divide into either two or four pieces. Roll out thinly, then put on the cold baking sheets. Spread the tomato sauce over the dough and scatter with the basil and mozzarella. Add any other toppings of your choice. Drizzle with olive oil and put the baking sheets in the oven on top of the preheated ones. Cook for 8–10 minutes until golden and crisp, then serve the pizza cut into wedges.

Lifesaver for your store cupboard
tomato sauce
For serving with grilled/broiled meats and fish, as a pizza topping, with pasta or gnocchi, as a soup base (add stock and cream), a dip or salsa with chilli, simmer **750g/1lb 10oz/3 cups canned chopped tomatoes, 3 tbsp olive oil, 2 crushed garlic cloves, 1 tsp caster/superfine sugar, 1 tsp balsamic vinegar, 2 tbsp chopped basil leaves** (optional), and a little **sea salt** and **freshly ground black pepper** in a pan for 30 minutes until rich and thick. Use straight away or cool and store in the refrigerator for up to a week. To keep, spoon into sterilized jars, seal loosely with a lid and put in a roasting pan lined with a folded dish towel and fill 2cm/¾in deep with hot water. Put in a preheated oven at 160°C/315°F/gas 2–3 for 25 minutes, then seal tightly. Store in a cool, dark place and use within 6 months. Once open, store in the refrigerator and use within 3 days.

There's no racing about and getting in a flap with this roast dinner – everything you need is cooked in one pan. If you are lucky enough to have any leftovers, then you must try the Roast Chicken Pies.

Simple Slow-roast Chicken Dinner

MAKES 2 adult and 2 kid-sized portions
PREPARATION TIME 15 minutes
COOKING TIME 3 hours

1.8kg/4lb free-range or organic chicken
40g/1½oz butter, softened
1 butternut squash, halved, peeled, deseeded and cut into wedges
2 large carrots, peeled and cut into large chunks
2–3 parsnips, peeled and cut into chunks (central core removed if tough)
1 garlic bulb, halved through the middle
2–3 rosemary, thyme or sage sprigs
500ml/17fl oz/2 cups chicken stock
125ml/4fl oz/½ cup white wine
1 tbsp cornflour/cornstarch
2 tbsp cream or crème fraîche (optional)
sea salt and freshly ground black pepper

1 Preheat the oven to 160°C/315°F/gas 2–3.

2 Put the chicken in a large roasting pan and smear the butter over the chicken and the base of the pan. Put the vegetables, garlic and herbs round the chicken. Pour over 125ml/4fl oz/½ cup of the stock and the wine. Season lightly with salt and pepper. Cover the pan with a piece of foil and roast for 1 hour. Remove the foil, baste the chicken and vegetables with the pan juices, turning the vegetables. Return to the oven and cook, uncovered, for a further 1 hour.

3 Increase the oven temperature to 220°C/425°F/gas 7. Baste the chicken and vegetables, then cook for 30 minutes until the chicken is golden and the juices from the chicken run clear when the thickest part of the thigh is pierced with a skewer.

4 Remove the chicken from the roasting pan and leave it to rest, loosely covered with foil. Return the pan to the oven for 15 minutes to crisp the vegetables. Transfer the vegetables to a serving plate.

5 Drain off the fat and put the roasting pan over a high heat. Add the remaining stock and any resting juices from the chicken and scrape any sticky residue from the base and sides of the pan. Stir 1 tbsp water into the cornflour/cornstarch, then stir this into the pan and bring to the boil. Cook for 2 minutes, stirring continuously. Finish by stirring in the cream, if you like. Carve the chicken and serve with the vegetables.

Leftovers make tasty pies
roast chicken pies

Use leftover cooked chicken, or any meat, and veg to make a pie. Blend **1 tbsp butter** and **1 tbsp flour** in a pan over a low heat, then whisk in **240ml/8fl oz/ scant 1 cup hot stock** until smooth. Simmer for a few minutes, then stir in **2 tbsp double/heavy cream**, **1 tsp mustard**, **a squeeze of lemon juice**, **2 tbsp chopped parsley leaves** and season with **sea salt** and **freshly ground black pepper**. Add **200g/7oz each of chunks of cooked meat and veg**. Divide between one large or two individual pie dishes. Roll out **250g/9oz puff pastry** and moisten the edges to seal to the top of the dishes. Cut a hole in the top and brush with **egg**, **milk** or **oil**. Put on a hot baking sheet and bake in a preheated oven at 200°C/400°F/gas 6 for 30 minutes until golden and piping hot.

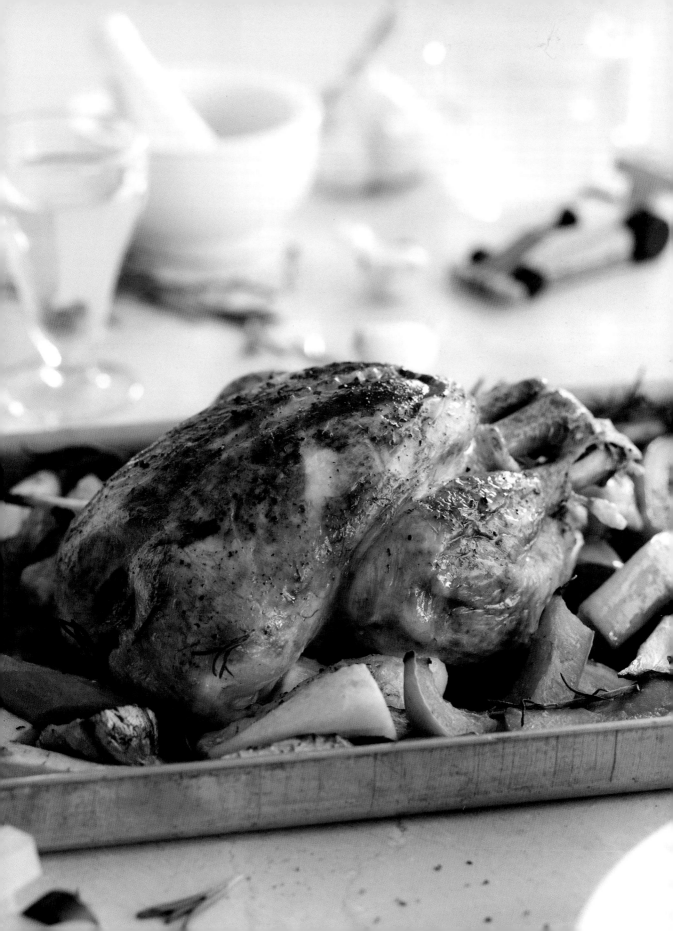

A delicious dish for busy families, it's a lovely thing to make on a Sunday night when you've been out for the day and need something to literally throw together. It's also just as delicious eaten cold as hot, so you can serve it the next day with a green salad and crusty bread.

Spanish(ish) Chicken Traybake

MAKES 2 adult and 2 kid-sized portions
PREPARATION TIME 15 minutes
COOKING TIME 1 hour

8–12 skinless chicken thighs (depending on their size)
2 red peppers, deseeded and cut into wedges
1 large onion, cut into 8 wedges
500g/1lb 2oz new potatoes, halved if large
4 garlic cloves, lightly crushed
1 lemon, cut into wedges
3 tbsp olive oil
20 thin slices of chorizo, halved
1 large handful of pitted green olives, plain or stuffed with pimiento or anchovies
150g/5½oz cherry or baby plum tomatoes
sea salt and freshly ground black pepper

1 Preheat the oven to 220°C/425°F/gas 7.

2 Put the chicken, red peppers, onion, potatoes, garlic, lemon and oil in a large roasting pan and toss everything together so it is coated in oil. Season lightly with salt and pepper. Put over a high heat on the hob and stir everything together for a couple of minutes to get some heat into it, then return to the oven to roast for 30 minutes, turning everything around in the pan halfway through.

3 Add the remaining ingredients, return to the oven and cook for a further 30 minutes, turning a couple of times to ensure even cooking, until everything is juicy, golden and delicious. The chicken juices from the chicken should run clear when the thickest part of the thigh is pierced with a skewer. Serve hot.

I love sweet potatoes to make a change from ordinary mashed potatoes, so here's an alternative bangers and mash dish. It's really easy and as an added incentive the washing up is minimal.

Sticky Sausages with Sweet Potatoes and Peppers

MAKES 2 adult and 2 kid-sized portions
PREPARATION TIME 15 minutes
COOKING TIME 1 hour

12 pork chipolata sausages
900g/2lb sweet potatoes, peeled and cut into wedges
2 red onions, cut into wedges
4 rosemary sprigs
2 red, yellow or orange peppers, deseeded and thickly sliced
3 tbsp olive oil
sea salt and freshly ground black pepper

FOR THE STICKY MIX
3 tbsp brown sugar
1 tbsp wholegrain mustard
1 tbsp white or red wine vinegar
1 tbsp orange or pineapple juice

1 Preheat the oven to 220°C/425°F/gas 7.

2 Put all the main ingredients, apart from the sticky mix, in a roasting pan and toss together. Roast for 30 minutes, giving everything a stir halfway through.

3 Stir together all the sticky mix ingredients and pour into the pan, giving everything a good stir so it is coated. Return to the oven and cook for a further 20–30 minutes, turning everything a couple of times until sticky and golden. Remove the rosemary sprigs and serve hot.

Leftovers for a filling salad
sausage and couscous salad

It is unlikely there will be any of this dish left over as it is exceptionally tasty and hard to resist. If there is, however, you can use it to make a salad to serve for your lunch the following day, either at home, or it makes a great packed lunch to take to school or work. Simply leave it to cool, then cut everything into bite-size pieces. Measure **100g/3½oz/heaped ½ cup couscous** into a bowl, pour over **100ml/3½fl oz/scant ½ cup boiling water** and stir together. Leave to stand for 10 minutes, stirring occasionally, until cool. Stir in a **dash of olive oil** and **a sprinkling of lemon juice**, then the **sausages** and you are ready to go.

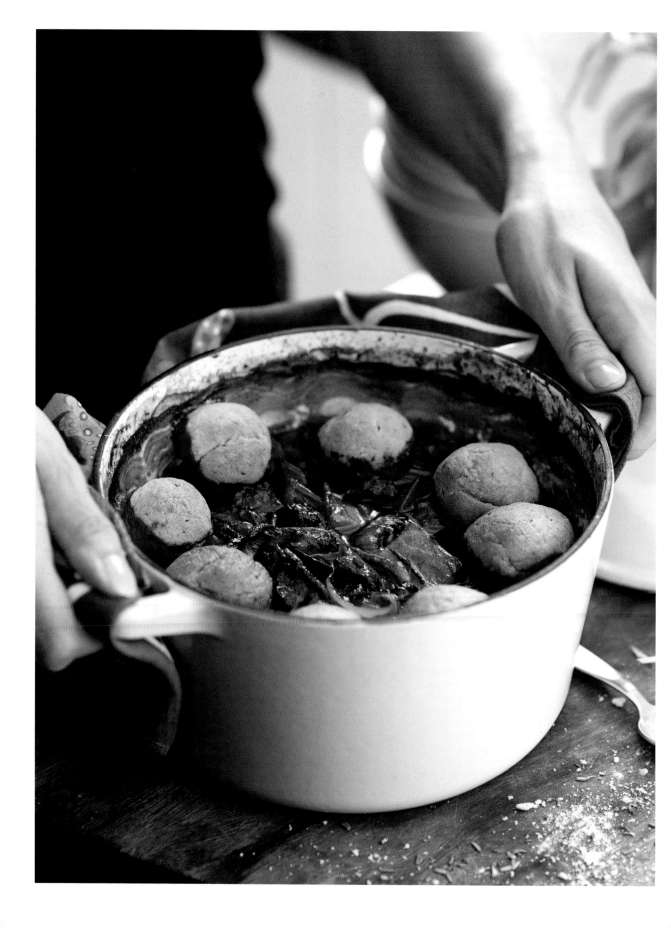

This hearty casserole is ideal to serve as an alternative to a roast when you've little time to prepare. Simply throw everything in a casserole dish, pop it in the oven and leave it to cook. The only other thing to do is whizz together the dumpling ingredients in a food processor and put on top of the casserole towards the end of its cooking time.

Lamb and Redcurrant Casserole with Rosemary Dumplings

MAKES 2 adult and 4 kid-sized portions
PREPARATION TIME 20 minutes
COOKING TIME 2½ hours

FOR THE CASSEROLE
750g/1lb 10oz lamb shoulder, diced
3 heaped tbsp plain/all-purpose flour
2 large onions, thickly sliced
½ swede/rutabaga, peeled and cut into
 bite-size pieces
2 celery stalks, sliced
2 carrots, peeled and sliced
3 tbsp redcurrant jelly
2 tbsp red wine vinegar
2 tsp Worcestershire sauce
2 tbsp tomato purée/paste
400ml/14fl oz/scant 1¾ cups red wine
200ml/7fl oz/scant 1 cup lamb or beef
 stock
sea salt and freshly ground black pepper
cabbage or curly kale, to serve

FOR THE DUMPLINGS
75g/2½oz/scant ⅔ cup self-raising flour,
 plus extra for dusting
75g/2½oz/heaped 1 cup fresh white
 breadcrumbs
75g/2½oz butter, diced
2 tsp Dijon mustard
1 tbsp finely chopped rosemary leaves
1 large egg, lightly beaten

1 Preheat the oven to 160°C/315°F/gas 2–3.

2 Put the lamb and flour in a bowl or large plastic freezer bag and toss well, making sure all the lamb is coated in the flour. Put the lamb and all the remaining casserole ingredients in a large flameproof casserole dish, mix well and bring to the boil over a high heat. Cover with a lid and bake for 2 hours until the sauce is thickening.

3 Meanwhile, make the dumplings. Put the flour, breadcrumbs and butter in a food processor and blitz until the mixture resembles breadcrumbs. Add the mustard, rosemary and egg, and season lightly with salt and pepper. Blitz briefly until the mixture forms a fairly moist dough. Using floured hands to stop the mixture sticking to you, divide the dough into 8 equal portions and shape them into balls.

4 After the casserole has been cooking for 2 hours, take it out of the oven and remove the lid. Put the dumplings on top of the lamb and sprinkle a few flakes of salt on top of each one. Return the dish to the oven, uncovered, for a further 30 minutes, until the dumplings are golden and the casserole is rich and thick. Serve the casserole just as it is or with some lovely buttery cabbage or curly kale.

Leftovers for something different
redcurrant lamb and green bean pie
Mix any **leftover casserole** with some **blanched green beans** and spoon into a large pie dish or individual dishes. Top with **puff** or **shortcrust pastry**, pierce a hole in the top and brush with a little **milk** or **egg yolk**. Bake in a preheated oven at 200°C/400°F/gas 5 for 25–30 minutes until golden.

The beauty of this recipe is that you can make the parcels small for younger children or big, using larger salmon fillets, for adults. You could also make it with filo/phyllo pastry, layering three sheets together by brushing with some melted butter.

Salmon Gone-in-a-puff Parcels

MAKES 2 adult and 2 kid-sized portions, depending on the size of the fillets
PREPARATION TIME 15 minutes
COOKING TIME 20 minutes

175g/6oz mascarpone or cream cheese
2 tbsp chopped dill or chives
1 tsp Dijon mustard
finely grated zest of 1 lemon
½ bunch spring onions/scallions, thinly sliced
4 salmon fillets, whatever size suits you all
375g/13oz ready-rolled puff pastry
1 egg yolk
1 tbsp milk
sea salt and freshly ground black pepper

TO SERVE
seasonal vegetables or salad
cooked potatoes, tossed in butter and chopped mint

1 Preheat the oven to 220°C/425°F/gas 7. Line a baking sheet with baking paper or use a non-stick baking sheet.

2 Mix together the mascarpone, dill, mustard, lemon zest and spring onions/scallions, and season lightly with salt and pepper. Spread over the top of the pieces of salmon.

3 Cut the pastry into four pieces big enough to wrap around each of the salmon fillets. Put the salmon fillets on the pastry and fold over the rest of the pastry to create a neat parcel. Trim any excess, if you need to. Cut a couple of holes in the top for any steam to escape when cooking, then put them on the prepared baking sheet. (You can cook straight them away or chill until needed.)

4 When ready to cook the parcels, mix together the egg yolk and milk to make an egg wash and brush it over the top of the parcels. Bake for 20 minutes until the fish is cooked through and the pastry is golden.

5 Serve hot with vegetables or salad, and cooked potatoes tossed in butter and chopped mint.

Lifesaver for the freezer
marinated five-spice salmon
If you've some fresh salmon fillets or steaks (or any other fish fillets for that matter) that you plan on freezing, coat them in a tasty marinade first. That way all you need to do is defrost the fish in the refrigerator on a day you want a quick and easy meal that's not out of a packet. For **1 fillet** or **steak**, mix together **½ tsp Chinese five-spice**, **2 tsp soy sauce** and **1 tbsp clear honey**. Add to a freezer bag along with the fish and seal tightly. Move the fish around to evenly coat in the marinade, label the bag and store in the freezer. Once the fish is defrosted, grill/broil, bake, fry or even barbecue until golden and cooked through. Add a **squeeze of lime** and serve with **noodles** or **rice** and **stir-fried vegetables**.

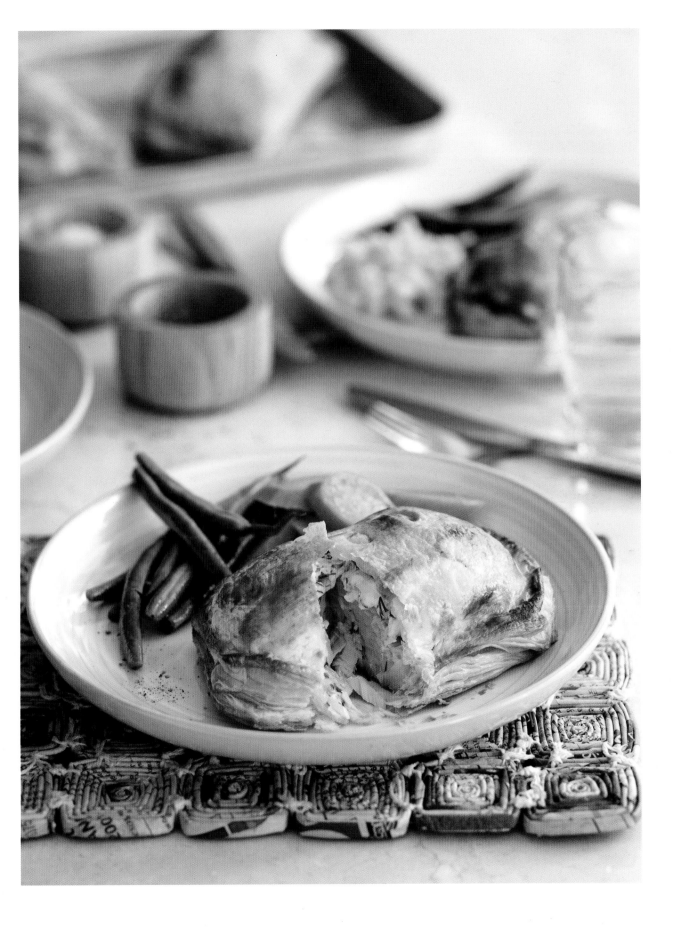

A humble sheet of puff or shortcrust pastry is a perfect canvas for a variety of toppings, depending on what you and your family like, are in the mood for, or you have sitting in the refrigerator. These recipes are favourites in my house, but feel free to be as creative as you like and come up with your own ideas for good flavour combinations.

Three Ways with Simple Savoury Tarts

EACH ONE MAKES 2 adult and 4 kid-sized portions
PREPARATION TIME 15 minutes
COOKING TIME 25 minutes

SMOKED SALMON AND LEEK TART

1 tbsp olive oil, plus extra for drizzling
25g/1oz butter
1 large leek, finely sliced
375g/13oz ready-rolled shortcrust or puff pastry
250g/9oz ricotta cheese
2 eggs, lightly beaten
2 garlic cloves, crushed
1 small handful of tarragon, chervil or parsley leaves, finely chopped
finely grated zest of 1 lemon
200g/7oz hot-smoked salmon or smoked trout, flaked
1 tbsp freshly grated Parmesan cheese
sea salt and freshly ground black pepper
green salad or vegetables, to serve

1 Preheat the oven to 200°C/400°F/gas 6 and line a baking sheet with baking paper.

2 Heat the oil and butter in a frying pan over a low heat, add the leek and cook gently for a few minutes until softened. Remove from the heat.

3 Lay the pastry on the prepared baking sheet, score a 2cm/¾in border with a sharp knife and prick the middle part of the pastry several times with a fork.

4 Mix together the ricotta, eggs, garlic, your chosen herb, salt and pepper. Spread over the pastry, inside the border, then top with the leeks, lemon zest and hot-smoked salmon. Finish by scattering over the Parmesan, add a drizzle of olive oil and brush the pastry edges with oil. Bake for 25 minutes until the pastry is golden and the filling softly set.

5 Serve hot with a green salad or vegetables.

SPINACH, PEPPER AND PINE NUT TART

200/7oz/1¾ cups frozen spinach,
  defrosted
250g/9oz ricotta cheese
2 eggs, lightly beaten
2 garlic cloves, crushed
¼ tsp freshly grated nutmeg
375g/13oz ready-rolled shortcrust or
  puff pastry
3 bottled or canned roasted red
  peppers, cut into strips
25g/1oz/¼ cup freshly grated Parmesan
  cheese
50g/1¼oz/⅓ cup pine nuts
olive oil, for drizzling
sea salt and freshly ground black pepper
green salad or vegetables, to serve

1 Preheat the oven to 200°C/400°F/gas 6 and line a baking sheet with baking paper.

2 Squeeze the excess water out of the spinach and mix together with the ricotta, eggs, garlic and nutmeg. Season lightly with salt and pepper.

3 Lay the pastry on the prepared baking sheet, score a 2cm/¾in border with a sharp knife and prick the middle part of the pastry several times with a fork. Spread the spinach and ricotta mixture over the pastry, inside the borders, and scatter over the red peppers, Parmesan and pine nuts. Drizzle with a little olive oil and brush the edges of the pastry with oil. Bake for 25 minutes until the pastry is golden and the filling softly set.

4 Serve hot with green salad or vegetables.

TOMATO, ASPARAGUS AND PARMA HAM TART

375g/13oz ready-rolled shortcrust or
  puff pastry
250g/9oz ricotta cheese
2 eggs
1 small handful of basil leaves, shredded
2 garlic cloves, crushed
25g/1oz/¼ cup freshly grated Parmesan
  cheese
12 tomatoes, halved
8–12 asparagus spears, cut into 5cm/2in
  lengths
6–8 slices of Parma ham
olive oil, for drizzling
sea salt and freshly ground black pepper
green salad or vegetables, to serve

1 Preheat the oven to 200°C/400°F/gas 6 and line a baking sheet with baking paper.

2 Lay the pastry on the prepared baking sheet, score a 2cm/¾in border with a sharp knife and prick the middle part of the pastry several times with a fork.

3 Mix together the ricotta, eggs, basil, garlic and half of the Parmesan. Season lightly with salt and pepper. Spread over the pastry, inside the border. Top with the tomatoes, asparagus and Parma ham, as rustic or neatly as you like. Scatter over the remaining Parmesan and drizzle with olive oil. Brush the edges of the pastry with oil. Bake for 25 minutes until the pastry is golden and the filling softly set.

4 Serve hot with green salad or vegetables.

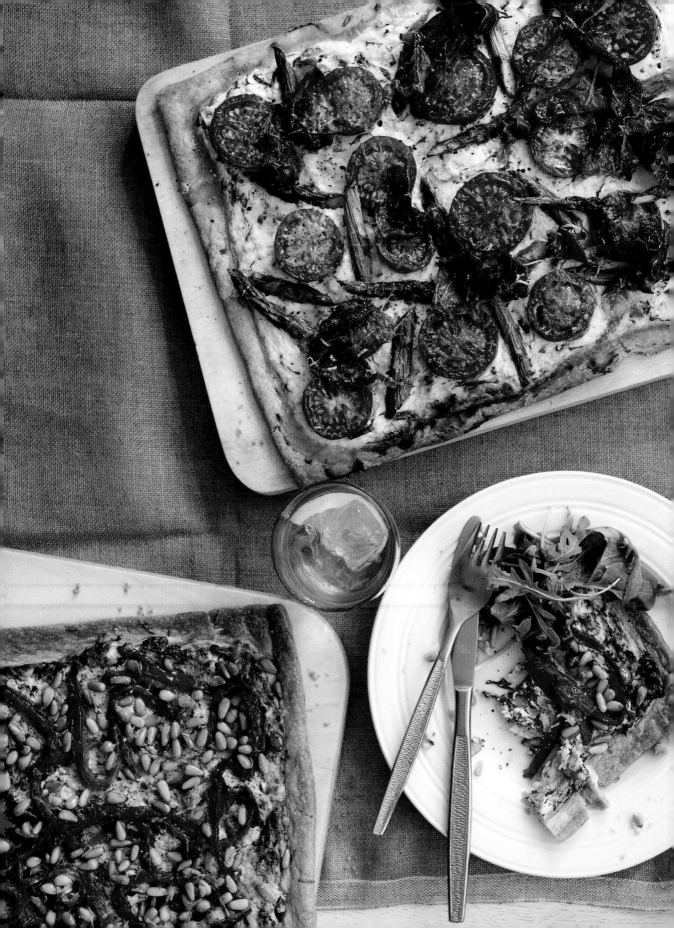

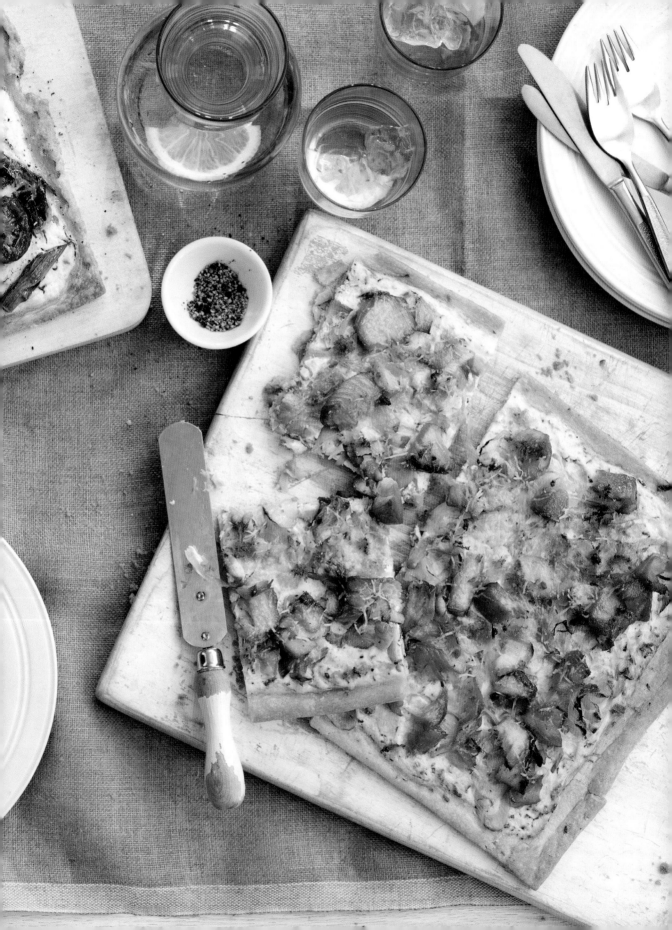

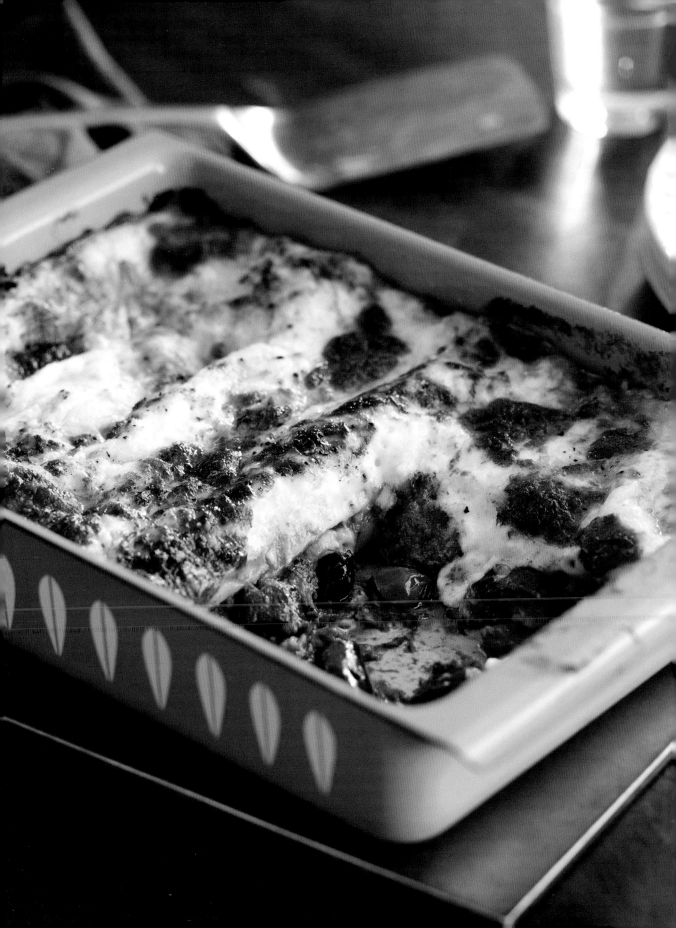

Whether you are a meat eater or not, this will go down a treat. It's hearty, nutritious and straightforward to prepare. I always make this quantity as it's a great lunch dish for an extended family, to serve the following day, or pop in the freezer if you have any left over. My bit of advice is to use fresh lasagne sheets, as you simply cut to fit your dish, rather than getting frustrated and in a mess by trying to snap dried sheets. No matter how hard you try, they never break where you want them to.

Rich Vegetable Lasagne

MAKES 4 adult and 4 kid-sized portions
PREPARATION TIME 25 minutes
COOKING TIME 1½ hours

2 red peppers, deseeded and cut into chunks
1 aubergine/eggplant, cut into chunks
2 courgettes/zucchini, cut into chunks
4 whole garlic cloves, unpeeled
3 tbsp olive oil
200g/7oz cherry tomatoes, halved
350ml/12fl oz/1½ cups passata/Italian sieved tomatoes with basil
2 tbsp red or green pesto
1 handful of chopped black olives (optional)
200g/7oz fresh lasagne sheets
125g/4½oz mozzarella, grated or torn into small pieces
25g/1oz/¼ cup freshly grated Parmesan cheese
sea salt and freshly ground black pepper

FOR THE BÉCHAMEL SAUCE
50g/1¾oz butter
1 bay leaf
50g/1¾oz/scant ½ cup plain/all-purpose flour
500ml/17fl oz/2 cups milk
¼ tsp freshly grated nutmeg

1 Preheat the oven to 200°C/400°F/gas 6.

2 Put the red peppers, aubergine/eggplant, courgettes/zucchini and garlic in a roasting pan and toss with the oil. Roast for 25 minutes. Add the cherry tomatoes and turn gently in the oil. Return to the oven and cook for a further 15–20 minutes until cooked through and lightly browned.

3 Meanwhile, to make the béchamel, melt the butter in a saucepan with the bay leaf over a medium heat. Once it is bubbling, stir in the flour and cook for a couple of minutes, stirring all the time. Gradually add the milk and bring to the boil, still stirring. Reduce the heat and stir until the sauce has thickened, then leave to simmer over a very low heat for 5 minutes, stirring occasionally. Remove the bay leaf, add the nutmeg and season lightly with salt and pepper.

4 Once the vegetables are cooked, remove the garlic cloves and squash the cooked garlic to a paste. Stir into the passata/Italian sieved tomatoes along with the pesto and olives, if using. Pour the passata/Italian sieved tomatoes into the vegetable pan, season lightly with salt and pepper and stir to combine.

5 Reduce the oven temperature to 180°C/350°F/gas 4.

6 Spoon one-third of the vegetable mixture into the base of a large ovenproof dish. Top with a layer of lasagne sheets, then drizzle over one-third of the béchamel sauce. Repeat so you have three layers of lasagne, finishing with the béchamel. Scatter over the mozzarella and Parmesan. (You can prepare the lasagne right up to this stage and chill until needed.) Put on a baking sheet and bake for 45 minutes until golden and bubbling. Leave to rest for 10 minutes, then serve.

An all-time favourite, I just had to include a sticky toffee pudding in the book, and my family love this banana version. The portions are deliberately generous to make sure there's plenty left over for the rest of the week.

Sticky Toffee and Banana Pudding

MAKES 2 adult and 2 kid-sized portions
PREPARATION TIME 15 minutes
COOKING TIME 30 minutes

FOR THE BANANA PUDDING
85g/3oz butter, softened, plus extra for greasing
250g/9oz dates, stoned and chopped
250ml/9fl oz/1 cup black tea
1 tsp bicarbonate of soda/baking soda
175g/6oz/heaped ¾ cup caster/superfine sugar
2 eggs, beaten
175g/6oz/scant 1½ cups self-raising flour
2 ripe bananas, peeled and mashed
1 teaspoon ground mixed spice
ice cream or shop-bought or Foolproof Home-made Custard (see page 128), to serve

FOR THE STICKY TOFFEE SAUCE
100g/3½oz/heaped ½ cup light brown sugar
100g/3½oz unsalted butter
125ml/4fl oz/½ cup double/heavy cream

1 Preheat the oven to 180°C/350°F/gas 4 and grease a 22cm/8½in square baking dish.

2 Put the dates and tea in a saucepan and bring to the boil. Cook for 3–4 minutes until soft, then stir in the bicarbonate of soda/baking soda.

3 Beat together the butter and caster/superfine sugar, using an electric mixer, until light and creamy. Stir in the eggs, flour, bananas, mixed spice and date mixture until well combined. Pour into the prepared baking dish and bake for 40–45 minutes until the top is just firm to the touch.

4 Meanwhile, to make the sauce, put the brown sugar, butter and cream in a saucepan over a low heat and cook gently until the sugar has dissolved and the sauce is a light toffee colour. (Both the pudding and sauce can be gently reheated and served within a few days. Alternatively, a slice of pudding can be popped into lunchboxes or enjoyed with your afternoon cuppa.)

5 Once cooked, pour the warm sticky toffee sauce over the pudding and serve with ice cream or custard.

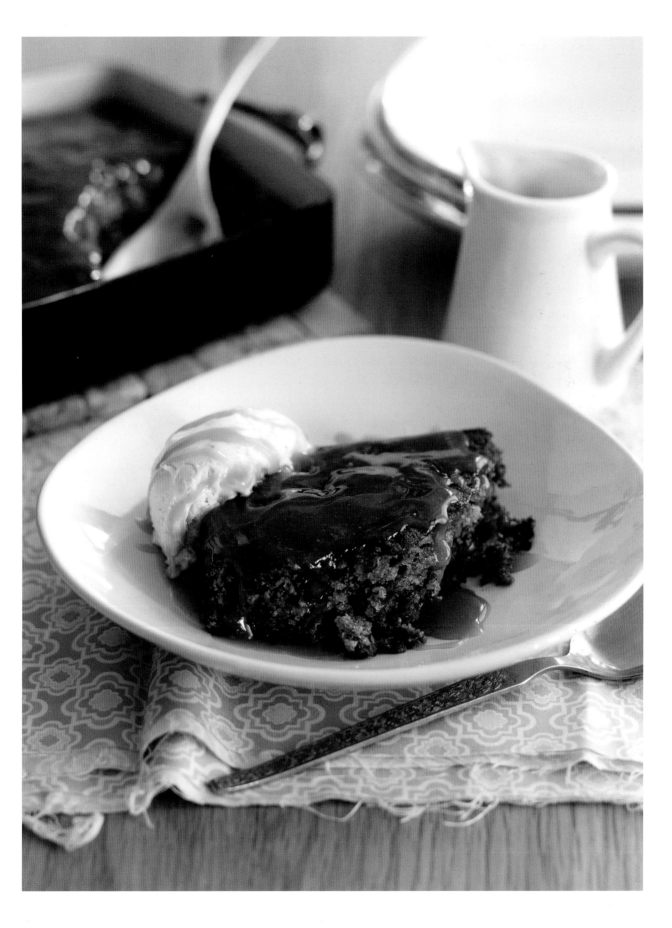

A household favourite when I was growing up, this is now fast becoming a favourite of my kids. Maybe this could become your Madhouse signature dish?

Saucy Chocolate Orange Pudding

MAKES 2 adult and 2 kid-sized portions
PREPARATION TIME 20 minutes
COOKING TIME 40 minutes

FOR THE CHOCOLATE AND ORANGE PUDDING
115g/4oz butter, softened, plus extra for greasing
115g/4oz/½ cup caster/superfine sugar
finely grated zest of 1 large orange
½ tsp vanilla extract
a pinch of salt
85g/3oz/⅔ cup self-raising flour
2 tbsp unsweetened cocoa powder
2 eggs
2 tbsp milk
cream or ice cream (optional), to serve

FOR THE CHOCOLATE SAUCE
115g/4oz/scant cup soft brown sugar
2 tbsp unsweetened cocoa powder

1 Preheat the oven to 190°C/375°F/gas 5 and grease a 1.2l/40fl oz/4¾ cup baking dish or pie dish with butter.

2 Beat together the butter, caster/superfine sugar, orange zest, vanilla extract and salt, using an electric mixer, until light and creamy. In a separate bowl, sift together the flour and unsweetened cocoa powder, then add one spoonful to the butter mixture along with 1 egg. Beat well, then repeat with the other egg. Finally, mix in the remaining flour and unsweetened cocoa powder along with the milk to give a soft dropping consistency. Transfer to the prepared dish and smooth the surface with a spatula.

3 Now for the wow factor. Mix together the soft brown sugar, unsweetened cocoa powder and 300ml/10½fl oz/scant 1¼ cups just-boiled water until the cocoa has dissolved. Pour over the top of the pudding, then bake for 40 minutes until springy to the touch.

4 Spoon the chocolate orange sponge into bowls, revealing the rich and delicious sauce at the bottom of the dish. Serve as it is or with cream or ice cream, if you like.

Leftovers for a sweet herb flavour
dill and orange butter
If you have used the orange zest, you'll obviously want a way to use up the juice. Put the **juice of 1 orange** in a small saucepan over a medium heat and cook until you have just 2 tbsp remaining. Beat into **125g/4½oz softened butter** with **1 tbsp chopped dill**. Season lightly with **sea salt**. Spoon onto a piece of baking paper and twist together the ends to form a long sausage shape. Store in the refrigerator for a few days and slice off individual pieces when needed. Use to flavour fish when steaming or baking, or add a slice on top of cooked fish to melt over the surface.

Need a quick pud to quite literally throw together to finish off your family meal before the kids race off and find better things to do than be sociable with their parents? All you need is some fruit (fresh or frozen), meringues and cream. Then add more madness and pimp it up with anything you can find in your baking cupboard.

Madhouse Mess

MAKES 2 adult and 2 kid-sized portions
PREPARATION TIME 10 minutes

300ml/10½fl oz/scant 1¼ cups double/
 heavy or whipping cream, or Greek
 yogurt, crème fraîche or ice cream
 (defrosted to a dolloping consistency)
3–4 meringue nests or 2–3 handfuls of
 mini meringues
300g/10½oz/2 cups soft fruit, cut into
 small pieces if necessary; virtually
 anything goes, such as fresh or frozen
 (defrosted) berries, bananas, ripe
 pears, canned fruit such as peaches,
 apricots, pears or cherries, grapes,
 mango etc.
2 tbsp jam, such as raspberry, strawberry
 or cherry (optional)

TO PIMP IT UP
choose your favourites from:
• chocolate chips
• cake sprinkles
• chocolate sweets
• mini marshmallows
• popping candy
• space dust
• or anything else your kids can
 get their hands on

1 Put the cream, or whatever you are using, in a large mixing bowl. If you are using cream, then whisk to form soft peaks. Crumble in the meringue, then throw in the fruit. Fold everything together using a large spoon, then swirl in the jam, if using – if the fruits you are using are quite sweet, the jam won't be necessary.

2 Spoon into dishes and, if you're pimping up your Madhouse Mess, scatter over your chosen treat and tuck in.

Ice cream in an instant – your kids will be amazed! Don't worry if you don't have frozen cherries, you can use frozen raspberries or berry mixes instead. You may need to add a little extra honey for sweetness. Alternatively, to make a banana ice cream, peel and chop four bananas. Freeze in a plastic freezer bag for a couple of hours, then use as below instead of the cherries.

Magic Ice Cream

EACH ONE MAKES 500ml/17fl oz/2 cups
PREPARATION TIME 5 minutes

CHERRY ICE CREAM

350g/12oz/2⅓ cups frozen pitted cherries
150ml/5fl oz/scant ⅔ cup shop-bought or Foolproof Home-made Custard (see page 128)
80ml/2½fl oz/⅓ cup double/heavy cream
2–3 tbsp clear honey

1 Put all the ingredients in a food processor and whizz until you have a soft, smooth, creamy ice cream.

2 Either serve straight away or transfer to a container with a lid and store in the freezer.

NUTTY BANANA AND CHOCOLATE ICE CREAM

4 ripe bananas, peeled, cut into chunks and pre-frozen
150ml/5fl oz/scant ⅔ cup shop-bought or Foolproof Home-made Chocolate Custard (see page 128)
80ml/2½fl oz/⅓ cup double/heavy cream
3 tbsp chocolate and hazelnut spread
chopped toasted hazelnuts, for sprinkling

1 Put all the ingredients except the chopped nuts in a food processor and whizz until you have a soft, smooth, creamy ice cream.

2 Either serve straight away scattered with chopped nuts or transfer to a container with a lid and store in the freezer.

MANGO ICE CREAM WITH COOL COCONUT SPRINKLES

350g/12oz frozen mango chunks
150ml/5fl oz/scant ⅔ cup shop-bought or Foolproof Home-made Custard (see page 128)
80ml/2½fl oz/⅓ cup double/heavy cream
2–3 tbsp clear honey

FOR THE SPRINKLES
a few handfuls of desiccated/dried shredded coconut
different coloured food colouring

1 For the sprinkles, put 1 handful of coconut in a freezer bag and add a drop of food colouring. Seal with air in the bag and shake like crazy until the coconut is coloured. Tip onto a plate to dry for a few minutes. Repeat with as many colours as you like.

2 To make the ice cream, put all the ingredients in a food processor and whizz until you have a soft, smooth, creamy ice cream.

3 Either serve straight away scattered with coloured coconut sprinkles or transfer to a container with a lid and store in the freezer. (Leftover sprinkles can be stored in an airtight container for weeks.)

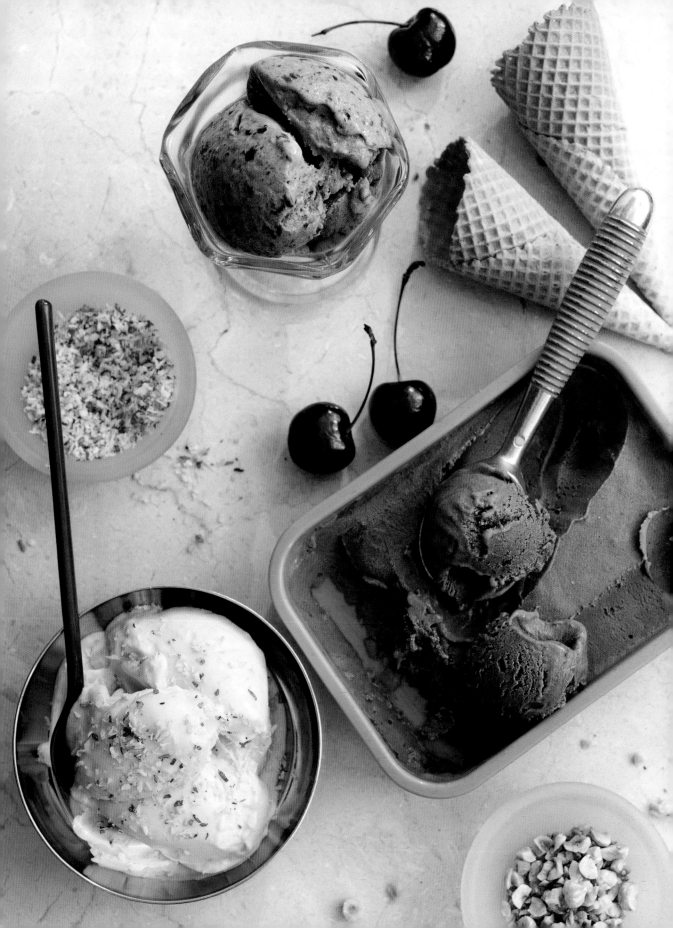

I've always wondered how to make fruit leather, partly due to my kids loving and also because buying it is expensive. I saw a recipe in the *River Cottage Handbook No.2, Preserves* by Pam Corbin, had a play around and came up with this. It's delicious, great to make with the children – and not bad for you either.

Blueberry and Apple Fruit Strips

MAKES about 20x30cm/8x12in sheet to cut into strips
PREPARATION TIME 10 minutes
COOKING TIME 30 minutes on the hob, then 6–8 hours on a very low heat in the oven

250g/9oz/1⅔ cups blueberries
250g/9oz Bramley cooking apples, peeled, cored and chopped
100g/3½oz clear honey
juice of ½ lemon
¼ tsp vanilla extract

1 Put all the ingredients in a saucepan and bring to the boil over a medium heat. Reduce the heat and leave to simmer for about 25–30 minutes until you have a thick purée, stirring occasionally.

2 When it is almost ready, preheat the oven to 70°C/150°F/gas ¼ and line a large baking sheet with baking paper (not greaseproof/waxed paper) or even a silicone sheet.

3 Press the purée through a sieve/fine-mesh strainer, pushing as much of the purée through as possible. Thinly spread the purée over the baking sheet to a rectangle about 20x30cm/8x12in as evenly as you can. Pop in the oven and leave for about 6–8 hours until the purée has firmed up and dried out.

4 Carefully peel the fruit strip away from the baking paper and hold it up to the light. It looks amazing! Cut it into strips and roll into coils. (The fruit strips can be kept for a couple of months in an airtight container.)

Never throw away over-ripe bananas again as it's so easy to make this tasty and quick-to-whizz-together loaf with them instead. You can leave out the ginger, if it's not your thing. If you don't have a loaf pan, make individual Banana and Ginger Muffins. Line a 12-hole muffin pan with paper muffin cases and spoon in the mixture. Reduce the baking time to 18–20 minutes until the muffins are golden and springy to the touch. Cool on a wire rack, then dust with icing/confectioners' sugar to serve.

Banana and Ginger Loaf

MAKES 900g/2lb loaf
PREPARATION TIME 10 minutes
COOKING TIME 1 hour

175g/6oz butter, softened, plus extra for greasing
2 really ripe bananas, peeled and roughly chopped
3 balls stem ginger, roughly chopped
2 eggs
175g/6oz/scant 1 cup soft light brown sugar
175g/6oz/scant 1½ cups self-raising flour
½ tsp vanilla extract
a pinch of salt
icing/confectioners' sugar, for dusting

1 Preheat the oven to 160°C/315°F/gas 2–3. Grease a 900g/2lb loaf pan with butter and line with baking paper.

2 Put all the ingredients in a food processor and whizz until smooth. Spoon into the prepared pan and smooth over the surface with the back of your spoon. Bake for 1 hour until the top is golden and the cake is cooked through. To test, insert a skewer into the centre. If the cake is cooked, the skewer will come out clean. If not, return the cake to the oven for a further 5–10 minutes.

3 Leave to cool in the pan for 10 minutes, then turn out and leave to cool on a wire rack. Dust with icing/confectioners' sugar and serve warm or cold.

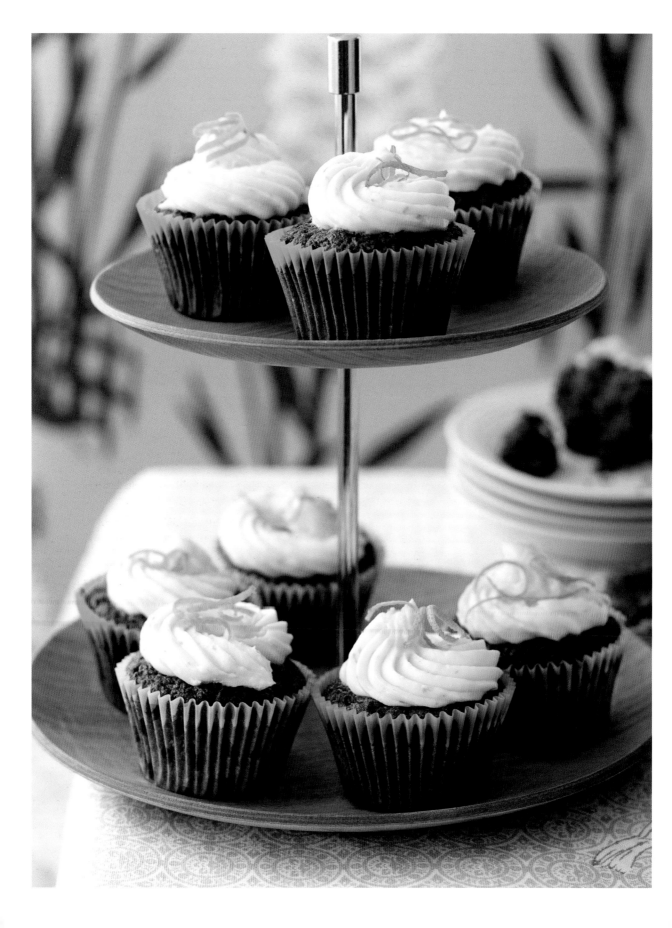

These delicious little cakes will keep easily for a few days in an airtight container in a cool place, and still be nice and moist. If you fancy making a large cake, grease and line two 18cm/7in round cake pans and divide the mixture evenly between them. Bake for 20–25 minutes.

Carrot Cupcakes with Cream Cheese Frosting

MAKES 12 cupcakes
PREPARATION TIME 20 minutes
COOKING TIME 20 minutes

FOR THE CARROT CUPCAKES
150ml/5fl oz/scant ⅔ cup rapeseed/ canola or sunflower oil
100g/3½oz/heaped ½ cup soft light brown sugar
2 eggs, lightly beaten
75g/2½oz golden/light corn syrup
175g/6oz/scant 1½ cups wholemeal or white self-raising flour
1 tsp ground cinnamon
¼ tsp ground allspice
½ tsp ground ginger
1 tsp bicarbonate of soda/baking soda
200g/7oz carrots, peeled and finely grated
75g/2½oz/scant ⅔ cup sultanas/golden raisins
25g/1oz/¼ cup desiccated/dried shredded coconut

FOR THE CREAM CHEESE FROSTING
100g/3½oz unsalted butter, at room temperature
100g/3½oz cream cheese
finely grated zest of 1 orange, plus extra to decorate
250g/9oz/2 cups icing/confectioners' sugar, sifted

1 Preheat the oven to 180°C/350°F/gas 4 and line a 12-hole cupcake pan with paper cupcake cases or lightly grease a silicone cupcake pan.

2 In a large bowl, whisk together the oil, sugar, eggs and golden/light corn syrup, using an electric mixer, until totally combined. Mix in all the remaining cake ingredients and spoon into the cupcake cases.

3 Bake for 20 minutes until nicely risen and firm but springy when lightly pressed. Leave to cool in the pan for 5 minutes, then transfer to a wire rack to cool.

4 To make the frosting, beat the butter until smooth, using an electric mixer. Add the cream cheese and orange zest and beat for another minute or so. Add half of the icing/confectioners' sugar and mix together on a low speed. Add the remaining icing/confectioners' sugar and mix until the icing has a light, creamy texture. Chill until needed.

5 When the cakes are completely cool, spread or pipe the frosting on top, sprinkle with extra orange zest and serve.

Lifesaver for a speedy cake
cream cheese frosting
The cream cheese frosting recipe freezes really well, so it is well worth making a double quantity and storing it in the freezer. Then, if you ever need to tart up a shop-bought cake, muffins or fairy cakes, you have a home-made frosting to hand. As an alternative to orange zest, you can flavour it with the **grated zest of 1 lemon**, **1 tsp ground cinnamon** or **ground ginger**, **seeds of 1 vanilla pod/bean**, or even colour it **pink** and add **a few drops of rose water**.

These muffins are fun, tasty (who doesn't love a marshmallow?) and irresistible when still warm from the oven. And if you do happen to have any left over a day or so later, don't throw them out as they can be used to make a delicious granola for breakfast.

Raspberry Marshmallow Muffins

MAKES 12 muffins
PREPARATION TIME 15 minutes
COOKING TIME 25 minutes

300g/10½oz/2⅓ cups self-raising flour
115g/4oz/½ cup caster/superfine sugar
150g/5½oz/1 cup fresh or defrosted, frozen raspberries
35g/1¼oz mini marshmallows
170ml/5½fl oz/⅔ cup milk
125g/4½oz butter, melted
1 egg, beaten

1 Preheat the oven to 180°C/350°F/gas 4 and line a 12-hole muffin pan with paper muffin cases or lightly grease a silicone muffin pan.

2 Put the flour, sugar, raspberries and marshmallows in a mixing bowl and lightly mix together so the raspberries are coated in flour. This will prevent the raspberries from sinking to the bottom of the muffins when they are cooking.

3 Mix together the milk, butter and egg, then gently mix into the flour mixture, creating a batter. Spoon into the muffin cases or pan and bake for 25 minutes until risen and golden.

4 Leave to cool in the pan for a few minutes, then transfer to a wire rack. Serve warm or cold. (If they are not all eaten up right away, store in an airtight container for a couple of days.)

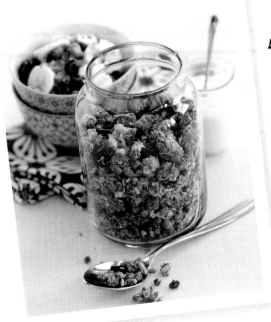

Leftovers for breakfast:
crunchy muffin granola

This couldn't be easier and makes a very yummy start to your day when eaten with milk or mixed with yogurt and fresh fruit for breakfast. Crumble **1 leftover muffin** into a bowl and then stir in **25g/1oz/¼ cup rolled oats, 1 tbsp sunflower seeds, 1 tbsp linseeds** (optional), **1 tbsp desiccated/dried shredded coconut** and **2 tbsp warmed clear honey**. Stir to combine, then put in a single layer on a baking sheet lined with baking paper. Cook in a preheated oven at 200°C/400°F/gas 6 for 10 minutes. Stir in **2 tbsp raisins, sultanas/golden raisins, dried cranberries** or **dried cherries** and return to the oven for 5–8 minutes until the granola is a deep gold. Leave to cool. Makes a generous adult portion or 2 smaller portions.

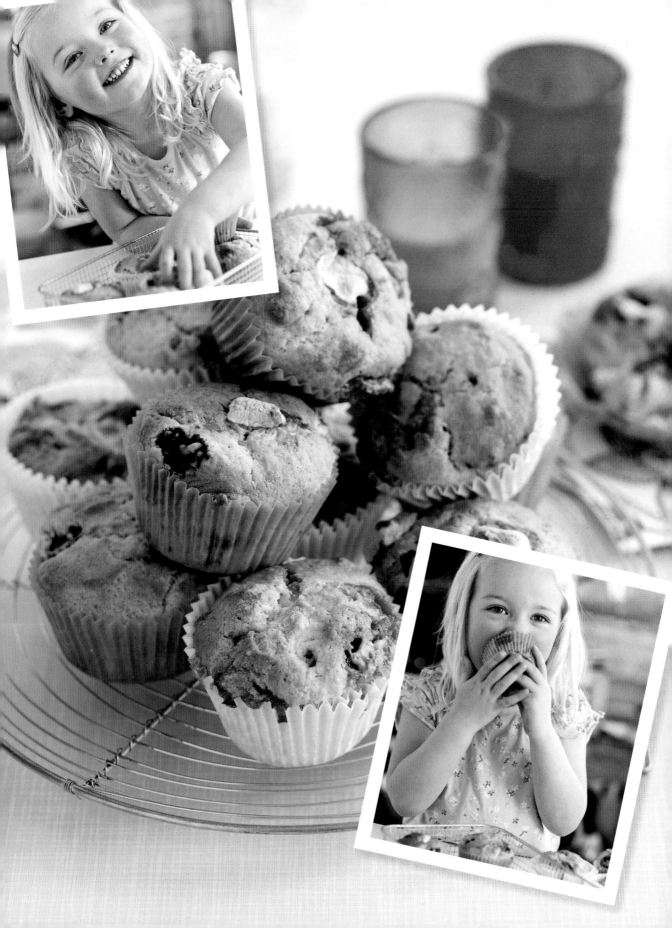

This makes a classic vanilla sponge that can be transformed into any number of things from a birthday cake to an impressive school cake sale masterpiece. Alternatively, if you want to keep it simple, fill with jam and whipped cream and dust the top with icing/confectioners' sugar. This will certainly give you a thumbs up from your grandma!

Classic Vanilla Sponge with Butter Icing

MAKES 20cm/8in cake
PREPARATION TIME 25 minutes
COOKING TIME 20 minutes

FOR THE CAKE
225g/8oz butter, softened, plus extra for greasing
225g/8oz/scant 2 cups self-raising flour, sifted, plus 1 tbsp extra for dusting
225g/8oz/scant 1 cup caster/superfine sugar
1 tsp vanilla extract
4 eggs

FOR THE BUTTER ICING
200g/7oz unsalted butter, softened
400g/14oz/scant 3¼ cups icing/ confectioners' sugar, sifted
3 tbsp milk
¼ tsp vanilla extract
food colouring (optional)

TO DECORATE
4–5 tbsp raspberry or strawberry jam
your choice of cake decorations, sprinkles or candles (be as elaborate as you wish)

1 Preheat the oven to 180°C/350°F/gas 4. Grease two 20cm/8 in cake pans with butter and lightly dust with flour.

2 In a large mixing bowl, beat together the butter, sugar and vanilla extract, using an electric mixer, for a good few minutes until the mixture is wonderfully light and fluffy. Beat in the eggs one at a time, adding a spoonful of the flour with each one to prevent the mixture from curdling. Fold in the remaining flour with a metal spoon until you have a soft, smooth cake batter.

3 Divide the mixture between the prepared pans and level the tops with a spatula. Make a slight dip in the centre to ensure that the cake is flat once cooked. Bake for about 20 minutes until the cakes spring back when pressed gently with a finger and are pale golden in colour.

4 Leave to cool in the pans for about 5 minutes, then transfer to a wire rack to cool completely.

5 To make the butter icing, beat together the butter, icing/confectioners' sugar, milk and vanilla extract, using an electric mixer, until it is really light and creamy. Add a few drops of food colouring, if you like, and beat it in well.

6 Sandwich the cakes together with a layer of jam and some butter icing, then use the rest of the butter icing to decorate the top and sides, along with whatever else you choose to use. Serve with a flourish.

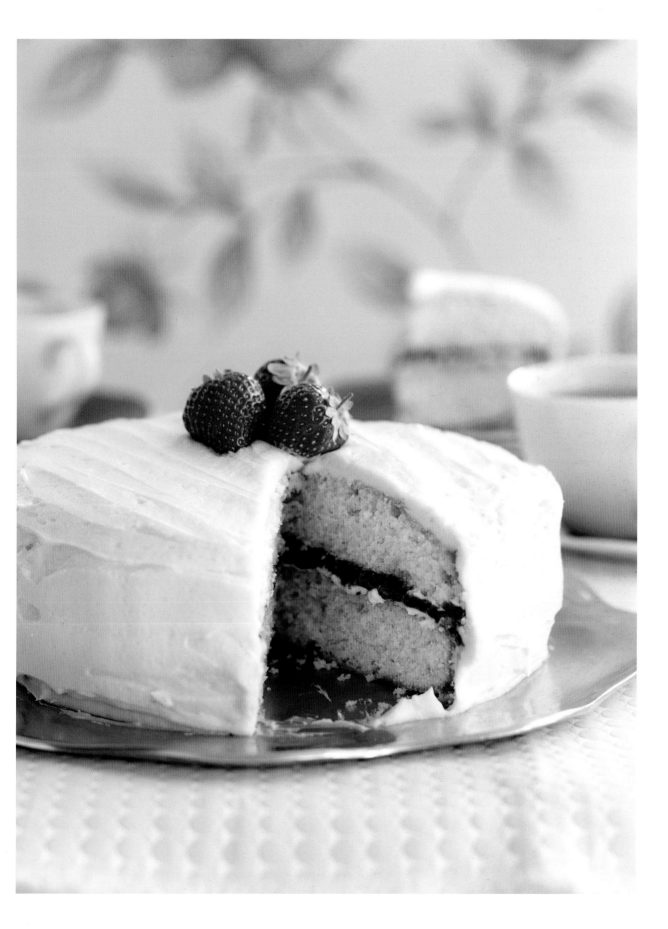

These little stunners don't take long to make and can act as lifesavers around the four o'clock mark on Saturday or Sunday with a cup of tea. Any left over will make a tasty treat during the week, as they will keep well for a good few days. You can also make them with raspberries, small strawberries or blackberries instead of blueberries. Frozen berries are perfect to use when fresh ones are out of season.

OMG Blueberry and Lemon Cakes

MAKES 12 cakes
PREPARATION TIME 15 minutes
COOKING TIME 15 minutes

275g/9¾oz/scant 2¼ cups icing/
  confectioners' sugar, sifted
75g/2½oz/scant ⅔ cup plain/all-purpose
  flour
50g/1¾oz/½ cup ground almonds
50g/1¾oz/½ cup desiccated/dried
  shredded coconut
½ tsp baking powder
150g/5½oz/1 cup blueberries
125g/4½oz unsalted butter, melted
finely grated zest of 1 large lemon
5 egg whites

1 Preheat the oven to 180°C/350°F/gas 4 and line a 12-hole muffin pan with paper muffin cases.

2 Mix together the icing/confectioners' sugar, flour, ground almonds, coconut, baking powder and blueberries. Then add the melted butter, lemon zest and egg whites. Mix until combined, then spoon into the muffin cases. Bake for 15 minutes until the cakes are golden and just springy to the touch in the middle.

3 Leave to cool slightly before removing from the pan. Serve warm or cold. (The cakes will keep in an airtight container for a few days and still remain really moist and yummy.)

How to make
foolproof home-made custard

Making your own custard is quite easy, and using a little cornflour/cornstarch will guarantee smooth results. To make 600ml/21fl oz/scant 2½ cups, put **570ml/20fl oz/scant 2⅓ cups milk** (or half milk, half double/heavy cream) and **¾ tsp vanilla extract** in a non-stick saucepan over a low heat and bring to simmering point. Meanwhile, whisk together **4 egg yolks**, **2 tsp cornflour/ cornstarch** and **40g/1½oz/scant ¼ cup caster/superfine sugar** until well blended. Gradually pour the hot milk into the eggs, whisking as you pour. Return the mixture to the pan and stir over a low heat until it has thickened, making sure it doesn't boil. Serve hot or pour into a bowl or jug, cover with cling film/plastic wrap (directly on the surface of the custard to prevent a skin forming) and cool. Chill in the refrigerator and use over the next 3 days.

P.S. If you fancied making Chocolate Custard, simply stir **50g/1¾oz dark chocolate**, 70% cocoa solids, into the hot custard until well combined.

This is one of those cake recipes that's perfect for a school cake sale or coffee morning as it's very easy and doesn't require any fancy finishing off. Nothing is wasted, either, as any leftover cake makes a lovely fruity base for a trifle and can even be made into Cake Pops (see page 220).

Lime and Orange Traybake

MAKES 16–20 squares
PREPARATION TIME 15 minutes
COOKING TIME 25 minutes

225g/8oz butter, softened, plus extra for greasing
225g/8oz/scant 1 cup caster/superfine sugar
grated zest and juice of 2 limes
grated zest and juice of 1 large orange
½ tsp vanilla extract
3 eggs
225g/8oz/heaped 1¾ cups self-raising flour
2 tbsp milk
4 tbsp granulated sugar

1 Preheat the oven to 180°C/350°F/gas 4. Grease a rectangular cake pan (about 20x30cm/8x12in) with butter and line with baking paper.

2 Beat together the caster/superfine sugar, butter, lime and orange zest and vanilla extract, using an electric mixer, until light and creamy. Beat in the eggs one at a time, adding a spoonful of the flour with each one to prevent the mixture from curdling. Mix in the remaining flour and the milk. Spoon into the prepared pan and level the surface with a spatula. Bake for 25 minutes, or until the sponge is golden and a skewer inserted into the centre comes out clean.

3 While the cake is cooking, put the lime and orange juice in a small saucepan over a medium heat. Bring to the boil, then boil to reduce to about 125ml/4fl oz/½ cup. Stir in the granulated sugar so it just starts to dissolve. As soon as the cake comes out of the oven, prick it several times over the top with a skewer or fork, then slowly spoon the lime and orange sugar all over the top, letting it soak into the cake.

4 Leave the cake to cool completely in the pan, then turn out and cut into pieces to serve.

Leftovers for a yummy trifle
citrus trifle

This is a refreshing trifle that uses up any traybake that has become a little dry. Put broken pieces of the leftover traybake in the bottom of individual dishes or a larger one to share. Pour over just enough **orange juice**, **orange liqueur** or **limoncello** to moisten the sponge. Top with a good portion of **sliced banana** and **cut-up orange**, **satsuma**, **mandarin** or **clementine segments**. Spoon over a thick layer of **shop-bought** or **Foolproof Home-made Custard** (see page 128) and then a layer of **whipped cream**. Finally swirl some lemon curd into the cream for a ripple effect and scatter with **a handful of toasted almonds** and **a little freshly grated lemon zest**.

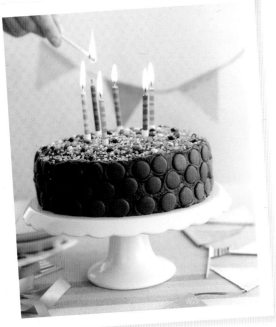

I have my grandma to thank for this recipe. She was always so organized, and she loved this cake because it could be made a day or so in advance but would still be lovely and moist when it was needed. It's ideal for birthday parties, when making a cake on the day of the party would send you into meltdown.

Moist Chocolate Cake with Chocolate Fudge Icing

MAKES 20cm/8in cake
PREPARATION TIME 25 minutes
COOKING TIME 35 minutes

FOR THE CAKE
150ml/5fl oz/scant ⅔ cup sunflower, groundnut or rapeseed/canola oil, plus extra for greasing
175g/6oz/scant 1½ cups self-raising flour, plus extra for dusting
4 tbsp unsweetened cocoa powder
1 tsp bicarbonate of soda/baking soda
1 tsp baking powder
130g/3½oz/heaped ⅔ cup caster/superfine sugar
2 tbsp golden/light corn syrup
2 eggs, lightly beaten
150ml/5fl oz/scant ⅔ cup milk

TO DECORATE
1½ tbsp unsweetened cocoa powder
100g/3½oz dark chocolate, 70% cocoa solids, broken into small pieces
150g/5½oz very soft butter
375g/13oz/3 cups icing/confectioners' sugar, sifted
½ tsp vanilla extract
a pinch of salt
4–5 tbsp raspberry or apricot jam
your choice of cake decorations, sprinkles or candles (be as elaborate as you wish)

1 Preheat the oven to 160°C/315°F/gas 2–3. Grease two 20cm/8in cake pans with oil and lightly dust with flour.

2 Sift the flour, cocoa powder, bicarbonate of soda/baking soda and baking powder into a large mixing bowl or food processor. Add the remaining cake ingredients and beat well to give a smooth, thick batter consistency. Divide the mixture evenly between the prepared cake pans and bake for 30–35 minutes until just firm to touch.

3 Leave to cool in the pans for 10 minutes, then turn out onto a wire rack to cool completely. (If you are planning a party, the cake will keep moist for a couple of days in an airtight container, either iced or plain.)

4 To make the icing, dissolve the cocoa powder in 3 tbsp boiling water and leave to one side. Put the chocolate in a large, heatproof bowl. Rest the bowl over a pan of gently simmering water, so that the bottom of the bowl does not touch the water. Stir occasionally until the chocolate has melted. (Or melt the chocolate gently in the microwave.)

5 In a large bowl, beat together the butter, icing/confectioners' sugar, vanilla extract and salt, using an electric mixer, until well combined, then add the melted chocolate and the unsweetened cocoa powder. Beat for a few minutes until thick and creamy.

6 Sandwich the cake together with the jam, then spread the chocolate fudge icing over the top and sides of the cake. Finish with any decorations and enjoy.

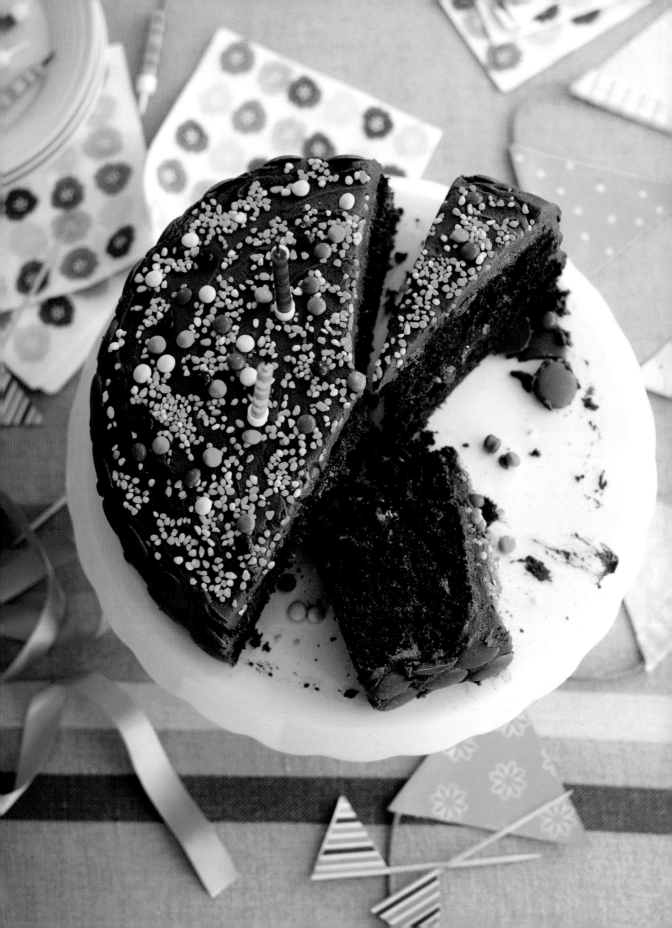

Freshly baked cookies still warm from the oven are virtually impossible to resist, so what could be better than having some cookie dough in the freezer, ready to create instant home-made cookies to enjoy with a glass of milk or a cuppa. These are light, crispy on the edges but slightly soft and chewy in the middle – otherwise known as perfect. For chocoholics, you can use chocolate chips or chunks instead of the fudge.

Fudge Freezer Cookies

MAKES 12–16 cookies
PREPARATION TIME 20 minutes
COOKING TIME 15 minutes

125g/4½oz butter, softened
100g/3½oz/heaped ½ cup soft light brown sugar
1 tbsp golden/light corn syrup
1 tsp vanilla extract
1 egg yolk
150g/5½oz/1¼ cups plain/all-purpose flour, plus extra for dusting
a pinch of salt
75g/2½oz small fudge chunks

1 Preheat the oven to 200°C/400°F/gas 6 and line a baking sheet with baking paper.

2 Beat together the butter, sugar and syrup, using an electric mixer, until light and creamy. Add the vanilla extract and egg yolk and whisk together briefly before sifting in the flour and salt and mixing until you have a smooth dough. Finally add the fudge chunks.

3 Using lightly floured hands to stop the mixture sticking to you, roll the dough into 12–16 balls. Put the cookies on the prepared baking sheet, making sure they are spread slightly apart. (If you don't want to bake all the cookies, put the remainder on a baking sheet lined with cling film/plastic wrap that will sit flat in your freezer. Leave in your freezer for about 1 hour for the dough to become solid, then peel it away from the cling film/plastic wrap. Put the uncooked cookies into a freezer bag or container to store for up to 2 months.)

4 Bake the freshly made cookies for about 10–12 minutes until they are just beginning to firm up but haven't become too dark around the edges. (If you bake the cookies from frozen, allow about 15 minutes.)

5 Leave to cool on the baking sheet for a couple of minutes, then transfer to a wire rack to cool completely before serving.

So quick to make and almost as quick to disappear, these nutty, crumbly cookies are a real family favourite. They are so easy to make, they are great to bake with the kids, too. You can use chunky or smooth peanut butter, whichever you prefer.

Peanut Butter and Jam Crumbly Cookies

MAKES 20 cookies
PREPARATION TIME 15 minutes
COOKING TIME 12 minutes

125g/4½oz butter, softened, plus extra
   for greasing
75g/2½oz/scant ⅓ cup caster/superfine
   sugar
75g/2½oz peanut butter
1 egg yolk
250g/9oz/2 cups plain/all-purpose flour
½ jar raspberry or strawberry jam

1 Preheat the oven to 180°C/350°F/gas 4. Grease two baking sheets with butter and line with baking paper.

2 Beat together the butter and sugar in a mixing bowl, using an electric mixer, until light and creamy. Mix in the peanut butter and egg yolk until combined, then mix in the flour to give a soft dough.

3 Take a heaped teaspoonful of the dough and roll into a ball. Put on the prepared baking sheets. Stick a thumb or finger into the middle of the dough ball to make an imprint deep enough to fill with about ½ tsp jam. Repeat using the remaining dough. Fill each imprint with jam, then bake for 10–12 minutes until they are lightly golden.

4 Leave to cool on the baking sheet for a couple of minutes, then transfer to a wire rack to cool completely before serving.

If it's raining and you need something to do to keep the kids occupied, these are perfect. They're also great if you need a gift for days like Mothering Sunday, Father's Day or a birthday as they can be any shape (such as a heart) and decorated accordingly (with more hearts … and a few kisses).

Get Creative Cut-out Cookies

MAKES about 30–40 cookies, depending on the size of cutters you use
PREPARATION TIME 15 minutes, plus 1 hour chilling
COOKING TIME 8 minutes

125g/4½oz butter, softened
150g/5½oz/heaped ⅔ cup caster/superfine sugar
1 egg
1 tbsp golden/light corn syrup
½ tsp vanilla extract
275g/9¾oz/scant 2¼ cups self-raising flour, plus extra for dusting
1 tsp baking powder
a pinch of salt
any icings or decorations you like

1 In a large bowl, beat together the butter and sugar, using an electric mixer, until light and creamy. Add the egg, golden/light corn syrup and vanilla extract, then mix in the flour, baking powder and salt, giving you a smooth dough. Split in half and wrap in cling film/plastic wrap. Pop in the refrigerator for about 1 hour to firm up.

2 Preheat the oven to 180°C/350°F/gas 4 and line one or two baking sheets with baking paper.

3 Dust the work surface and rolling pin with flour, then roll the dough to about 5mm/¼in thick. Cut out whatever shapes you like using a cookie cutter and put them on the prepared baking sheets. They can sit relatively close to each other, as they don't tend to spread during cooking. If you wanted to pierce a hole in the cookies to thread ribbon through, do this now, using the tip of a skewer. Re-roll the trimmings as much as you need to, to get as many cookies as possible.

4 Bake for 8 minutes, or until nicely golden. Leave to cool on the sheet.

5 Once cold, they can be left plain or decorated with any icings or decorations you like. (Undecorated cookies are best stored in an airtight container.)

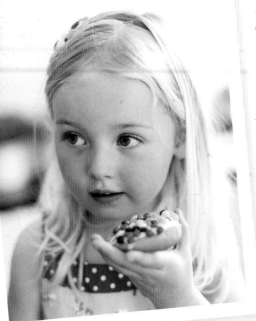

Lifesaver for teatime
cookie dough
If you don't want to cook loads of cookies all at once, it still makes sense to make this quantity of dough as you'll then have a Lifesaver when you need to magic a few cookies if the children bring a friend home to tea, or they just need something to amuse them. Wrap and label the dough. It will keep in the refrigerator for up to 5 days, or in the freezer for up to 3 months, then defrost, roll out and cook another day.

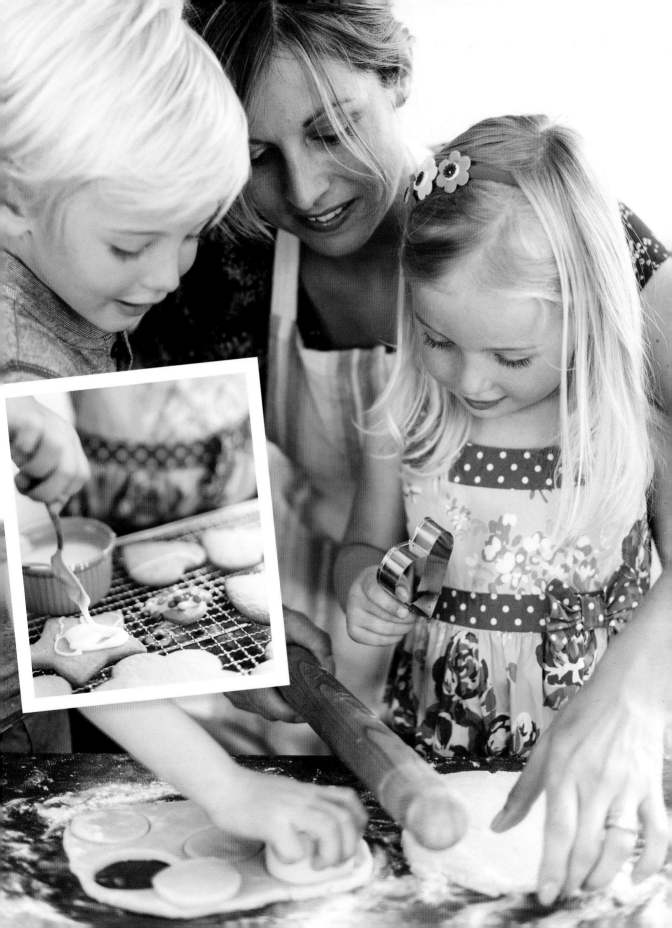

These work quite well in my house as a bribe: 'If you … get in the bath / get dressed / eat your tea / do your homework … you can have one of my flapjacks.' They even work on my husband.

Flap-free Flapjacks

MAKES 16 flapjacks
PREPARATION TIME 10 minutes
COOKING TIME 40 minutes

125g/4½oz butter, plus extra for greasing
140g/5oz/¾ cup soft light brown sugar
2 tbsp golden/light corn syrup
finely grated zest of 1 orange
175g/6oz/1¾ cups rolled oats
140g/5oz/1¼ cups dried fruit, such as raisins, sultanas/golden raisins, cherries, cranberries, chopped apricots, mango, apple, figs, prunes, dates
4 tbsp linseeds (in an attempt to be healthy!) (optional)

1 Preheat the oven to 160°C/315°F/gas 2–3. Grease a 20cm/8in square baking pan with butter and line with baking paper.

2 Put the butter, sugar, golden/light corn syrup and orange zest in a small pan over a low heat and gently melt together. Put the oats, dried fruit and linseeds, if using, in a bowl and pour in the melted butter and sugar mixture. Mix well to combine, then tip into the prepared pan. Press into the edges and flatten out with the back of a spoon.

3 Bake for 35–40 minutes until golden. Leave to cool in the pan for a few minutes, then turn out, cut into pieces and serve.

Leftovers with fruit, yogurt and spice
apple flapjack pots
The flapjack will keep for up to 4 days in an airtight container. Rather than eating it as a snack, break it into smaller pieces and scatter over Greek yogurt and fresh fruit as a breakfast treat or dessert. If you fancy a big boost of energy to start your day, or a delicious sweet treat at the end of a meal, a single piece of flapjack can go a long way. Another option is to make Apple Flapjack Pots as a great little dessert for the kids – or for you, as this makes an individual portion. Break **1 piece of flapjack** into small pieces and make alternate layers of **stewed apple** or **pear**, **Greek yogurt** mixed with **a pinch of ground cinnamon** and the flapjack in a glass or small dish. Finish with flapjack and enjoy.

A very naughty but nice treat, this is great for kids to make and give as little gifts. You can pack them in little boxes or cellophane bags tied with a piece of ribbon. (But do make extra and keep a few back to share.) You'll get the best flavour if you use chocolate with over 70 per cent cocoa solids; avoid cheap imitations.

Chocolate Bombs

MAKES 28 bombs
PREPARATION TIME 20 minutes, plus up
  to 1 hour chilling

175g/6oz dark chocolate, 70% cocoa
  solids, broken into small pieces
50g/1¾oz butter
2 tbsp golden/light corn syrup
150g/5½oz plain biscuits/cookies
150g/5½oz/1 cup glacé cherries

1 Put the chocolate, butter and syrup in a large heatproof bowl. Rest the bowl over a pan of gently simmering water, making sure that the bottom of the bowl does not touch the water. Stir occasionally until the chocolate has melted. (Alternatively, you can melt the ingredients gently in the microwave.)

2 Meanwhile, finely crush the biscuits/cookies, either in a freezer bag by bashing with a rolling pin, or in a food processor.

3 Rinse the cherries in a sieve/fine-mesh strainer and pat dry, then put on a chopping board. (Doing this will take away the stickiness.) Chop the cherries into small dice and add to the chocolate with 125g/4½oz of the crushed biscuits. Put in the refrigerator to firm up for 30 minutes–1 hour.

4 Take heaped teaspoonfuls at a time and roll into little balls or bombs. Roll in the reserved cookie crumbs to coat evenly, and repeat until all the chocolate mixture has been used up.

5 Once made, these will last for a couple of weeks in the refrigerator.

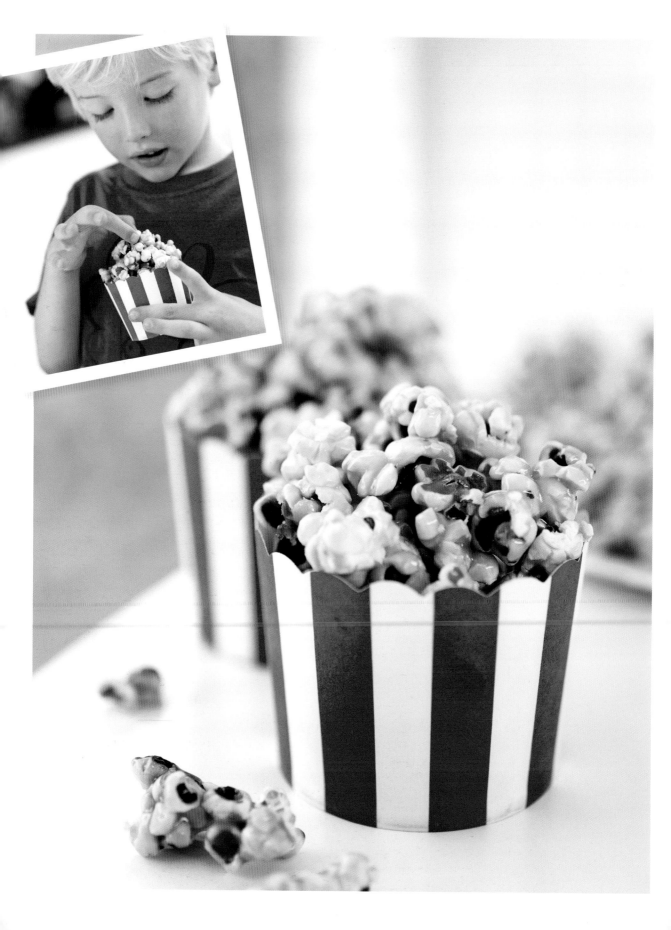

Weekends are all about having fun, and when it's cold and wet outside there's nothing my kids love more than chilling out and watching films. To give them a real treat, we'll make this super tasty popcorn to tuck into while they watch. It makes enough for you to enjoy, too, if you can spare a couple of hours to relax.

Sticky Toffee Popcorn

MAKES 4–8 portions
PREPARATION TIME 5 minutes, plus
   15 minutes cooling
COOKING TIME 5 minutes

1 tbsp sunflower oil
50g/1¾oz popping corn
40g/1½oz salted butter
40g/1½oz/¼ cup light muscovado sugar
2 tbsp golden/light corn syrup

1 Line a baking sheet with baking paper.

2 Heat the oil in a large saucepan over a medium-high heat. Add the corn and swirl the pan around to coat the corn in the oil. Cover with a tight-fitting lid. Reduce the heat to low and leave the pan for a few minutes until the popping has stopped, then remove it from the heat.

3 Meanwhile, put the butter, sugar and syrup in a separate pan over a low heat until the butter has melted. Increase the heat to medium and let the mixture bubble for 2 minutes. Pour over the popcorn and stir well to coat.

4 Spread the popcorn over the prepared baking sheet and leave to cool for about 15 minutes in a cool place (not the refrigerator) before serving.

Leftovers go savoury
cheese and onion popcorn
If you have leftover **popping corn**, you can make some savoury popcorn. Put it in a large pan, following the method above. In a separate pan over a low heat, melt **40g/1½oz butter**. Stir in **1 tsp onion salt** and remove from the heat. Pour the salted butter over the popcorn and scatter over **50g/1¾oz/⅓ cup finely grated Parmesan cheese**. Put the lid on the pan and shake it vigorously to coat the popcorn in the flavoured butter. Serve warm or cold.

This Lebanese-inspired recipe can be served as a starter with some warmed pitta bread (my favourite) or as part of a *maza* selection (the Lebanese equivalent of mezze), such as hummus, pickled chillies, stuffed vine leaves, bulghar wheat salad and olives.

Sautéed Chicken Livers with Pomegranate Molasses and Garlic

MAKES 2 adult portions
PREPARATION TIME 5 minutes
COOKING TIME 10 minutes

150g/5½oz chicken livers
1 tbsp plain/all-purpose flour
1 tbsp olive oil
about 1 tbsp butter
2 garlic cloves, finely chopped
2 tbsp pomegranate molasses
1 tbsp chopped flat-leaf parsley leaves
sea salt and freshly ground black pepper
toasted pitta bread, to serve

1 Pick over the chicken livers and trim off any fatty bits and sinew. Pat dry with paper towels. Season the flour lightly with salt and pepper, then toss with the livers so they are lightly coated in the flour.

2 Heat the oil in a frying pan over a high heat, add the livers and fry for 5–6 minutes until the outsides are crisp but the middles still a little pink (not raw) inside.

3 Add the butter and, when bubbling, throw in the garlic and cook for about 30 seconds. Add the pomegranate molasses and 1 tbsp water. Turn the livers in the pan so they are coated in the bubbling, sticky sauce. Stir in the parsley and season lightly with salt and pepper.

4 Serve with toasted pitta bread to mop up the sauce.

Leftovers for an aperitif
vodka, pomegranate and soda

The pomegranate molasses is really tasty made into a refreshing pre-dinner drink. Pour **1 tbsp pomegranate molasses** into a tall glass and add a **double or single shot of vodka (2–3 tbsp)**. Add a few **ice cubes** and a **good squeeze of lime** and stir around. Top up with **soda water**. Garnish with **pomegranate seeds** and **mint leaves**.

Serve this alone as a starter or as part of a tapas selection – with olives, cured hams, Manchego cheese, marinated anchovies, tortilla or your favourite antipasti. Double up on the prawns/shrimp if you don't have chorizo, or you could add a few squid rings.

Spanish Prawns with Sherry and Chorizo

MAKES 2 adult portions
PREPARATION TIME 10 minutes
COOKING TIME 15 minutes

2 tbsp olive oil
125g/4½ oz ready-to-cook chorizo
  sausage, cut into 1cm/½in thick slices
2 garlic cloves, crushed
125g/4½oz raw, peeled tiger prawns/
  jumbo shrimp
80ml/2½fl oz/⅓ cup dry sherry
200g/7oz/scant 1 cup canned chopped
  tomatoes or passata/Italian sieved
  tomatoes
1 bottled or canned roasted red pepper,
  sliced into strips
1 tsp sherry vinegar
a pinch of dried chilli/hot pepper flakes
1 small handful of flat-leaf parsley
  leaves, chopped
sea salt and freshly ground black pepper
crusty bread, to serve

1 Heat a frying pan over a medium heat. Add the oil and then add the chorizo. Cook for about 5 minutes until the sausage is cooked through and has released lots of rich, red oil.

2 Add the garlic and prawns/shrimp and cook for a further couple of minutes until the prawns/shrimp turn pink.

3 Add the sherry, tomatoes, red pepper, sherry vinegar and chilli/hot pepper flakes. Season lightly with salt and pepper. Increase the heat and cook for 4–5 minutes.

4 Stir in the parsley and serve with some crusty bread.

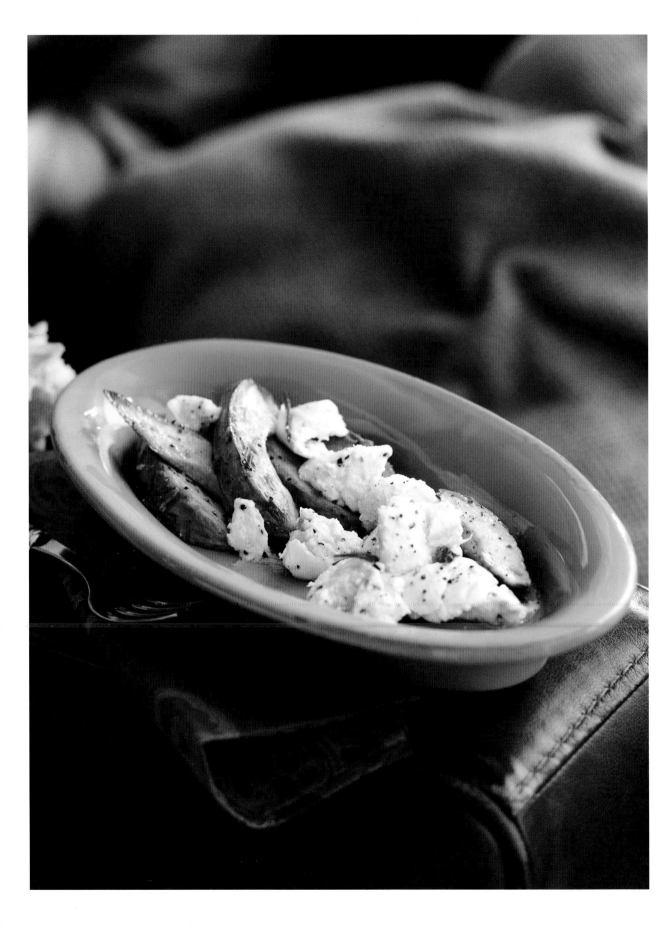

Create this delightful combination of flavours to serve with warm focaccia or ciabatta as a sophisticated starter, and treat yourself to a chilled glass of your favourite white wine as the perfect partner.

Chilli and Lemon Mozzarella with Pan-fried Avocado

MAKES 2 adult portions
PREPARATION TIME 10 minutes, plus 15–30 minutes marinating (optional)
COOKING TIME 5 minutes

125g/4½oz buffalo mozzarella, torn into pieces
grated zest and juice of ½ small lemon
½ red chilli, deseeded and finely sliced
2 tbsp extra virgin olive oil, plus extra for frying and drizzling
1 ripe avocado
sea salt and freshly ground black pepper

1 Put the mozzarella in a shallow non-metallic bowl. Mix together the lemon zest, juice, chilli and extra virgin olive oil. Season lightly with salt and pepper and pour over the mozzarella. Ideally, cover and leave to marinate in the refrigerator for 15–30 minutes.

2 To cook the avocado, cut in half and remove the pit. Peel away the skin and cut the flesh into slices about 1cm/½in thick. Heat a good drizzle of olive oil in a frying pan over a medium heat, add the avocado and fry for 1–2 minutes each side until lovely and golden. Remove from the pan, drizzle with extra virgin olive oil and season with salt and plenty of freshly ground black pepper.

3 Serve hot, with the marinated mozzarella and a lovely glass of chilled white wine.

Leftovers for snacks
mozzarella croque monsieur
If you have some marinated mozzarella and avocado (raw or pan-fried) left over, they are delicious made into a Italian-style Croque Monsieur. For a single portion, butter both sides of **2 pieces of bread**. Scatter small pieces of the **mozzarella** and **thinly sliced avocado** onto one piece of bread. Lay a piece of **ham** or **Parma ham** on top, then cover with the remaining piece of bread. Press down firmly. Heat a good **drizzle of olive oil** in a frying pan over a medium heat, add the sandwich and fry for 1–2 minutes on each side until the cheese is melting and the bread is toasted and golden. Serve hot.

Choose whatever flavoured sausages you like for this substantial main-course dish. I like using Toulouse, garlic and herb or venison. Dried Puy lentils work just as well but you'll need to cook for a little longer. Use 125g/4½oz/⅔ cup dried Puy lentils and add to the pan along with 150ml/5fl oz/scant ⅔ cup stock. Cook as in the recipe, but simmer for 45 minutes not 15 minutes.

Red Wine Sausages with Puy Lentils

MAKES 2 adult portions
PREPARATION TIME 10 minutes
COOKING TIME 45 minutes

1 tbsp olive oil
6 sausages
1 small red onion, finely sliced
½ large or 1 small red pepper, deseeded and finely sliced
250ml/9fl oz/1 cup red wine
1–2 oregano, thyme or rosemary sprigs (optional)
250g/9oz/1¼ cups ready-to-eat Puy lentils
200g/7oz/scant 1 cup canned chopped tomatoes
100g/3½oz baby or young spinach leaves
sea salt and freshly ground black pepper

1 Heat the oil in a deep frying pan over a medium heat, add the sausages and fry for 10–15 minutes until they are evenly browned. Remove from the pan and leave to one side.

2 Add the onion and red pepper to the pan and fry for 5–8 minutes until they are softened and the onion is becoming golden. Return the sausages to the pan. Add the red wine and the herb sprigs, if using. Bring to the boil and cook for a couple of minutes. Stir in the lentils and tomatoes. Bring to the boil, then reduce the heat, cover with a lid and leave to simmer gently for 15 minutes.

3 Remove the lid, stir in the spinach until it has wilted and heated through, then season lightly with salt and pepper.

4 Spoon the lentils into two bowls or deep plates, top with the sausages and spoon over any cooking liquid to serve.

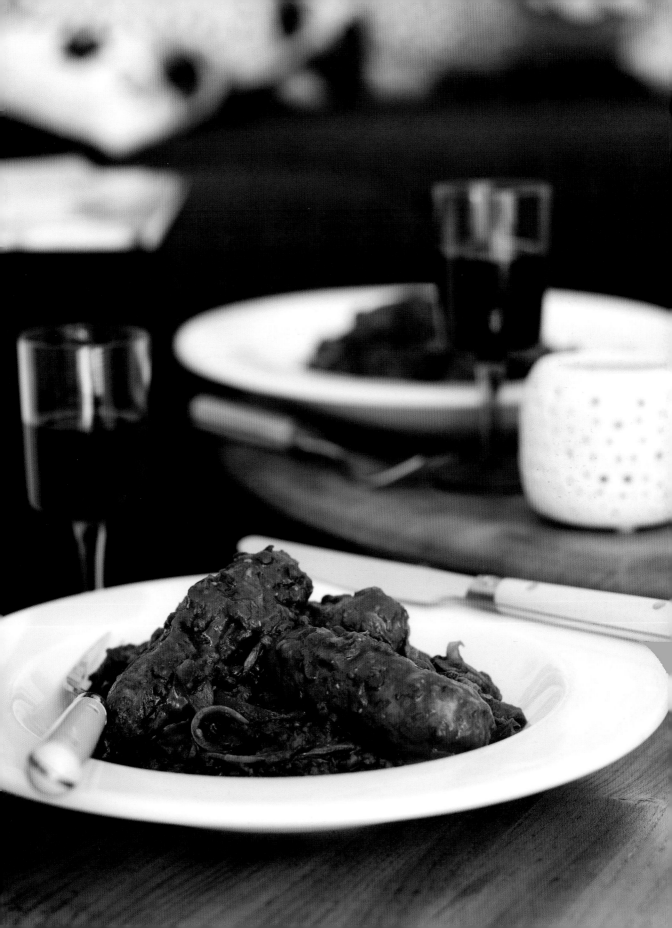

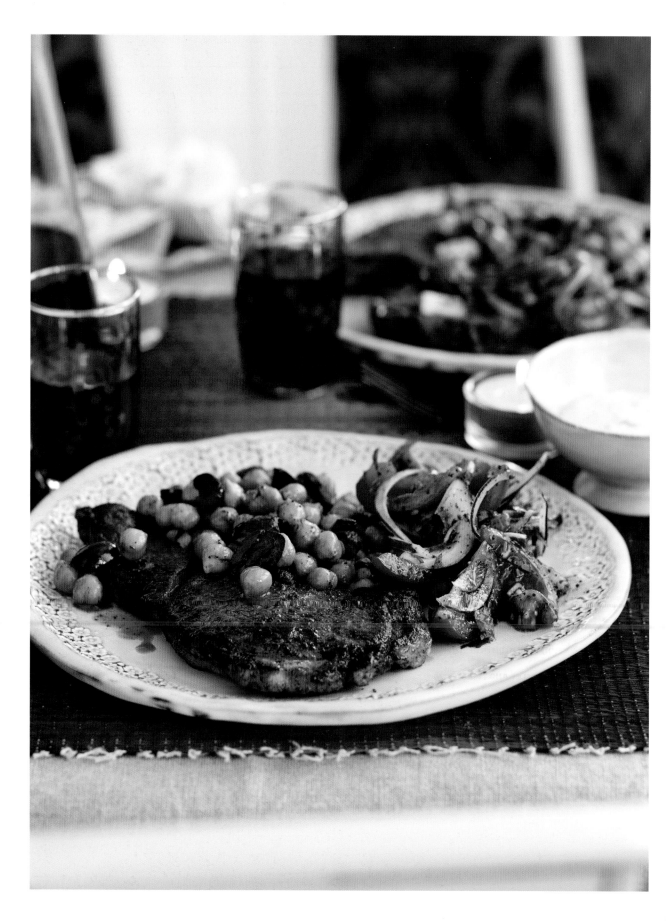

This Middle Eastern-inspired main course dish has spicy lamb steaks complemented by a fresh salad with a lemony tang. Try to cook the lamb so that it is still slightly pink in the centre. Sumac is a tart, acidic berry that's ground to a reddish-coloured powder and used widely in Middle Eastern cooking. It's usually found in the dried spice sections in supermarkets, so next time you see some, grab a jar. It adds a delicious tangy, lemony flavour to meats, fish, salads, hummus, rice dishes and much more. If you don't have any, replace it with a good squeeze of lemon juice.

Spiced Lamb and Chickpeas with Sumac, Parsley and Tomato Salad

MAKES 2 adult portions
PREPARATION TIME 15 minutes
COOKING TIME 10 minutes

FOR THE SPICED LAMB
2 lamb leg steaks (bone in, if possible, for a better flavour)
2 tbsp olive oil
1 tsp ground cumin
½ tsp paprika
½ tsp chilli powder
240g/8½oz canned chickpeas/ garbanzos, drained
130g/4½oz/1 cup black kalamata olives, halved and pitted
60ml/2fl oz/¼ cup white wine or chicken stock
sea salt and freshly ground black pepper

FOR THE SUMAC, PARSLEY AND TOMATO SALAD
3 ripe tomatoes, cut into wedges
½ red onion, finely sliced
1 small handful of flat-leaf parsley leaves, roughly chopped
1 tsp sumac
1 tbsp extra virgin olive oil

TO SERVE
3 tbsp Greek yogurt mixed with 1 tbsp chopped mint leaves
grilled/broiled flatbread or pitta bread (optional)

1 Put the lamb in a flat dish and rub in 1 tbsp of the olive oil along with the cumin, paprika and chilli powder. Leave to one side while you prepare the salad.

2 Heat the remaining olive oil in a frying pan over a medium heat, add the lamb steaks and fry for 2–3 minutes on each side until golden and still slightly soft to the touch. This will give you a medium finish. Cook for a shorter or longer time so the meat is cooked to your taste. Remove from the pan and leave to rest.

3 Add the chickpeas/garbanzos and olives to the pan and toss around for a couple of minutes to heat through. Add the wine, bring to the boil and boil for 30 seconds. Season lightly with salt and pepper, then pour in any of the lamb resting juices.

4 Meanwhile, toss together the salad ingredients and season with salt and pepper.

5 Put the lamb steaks, chickpeas/garbanzos and salad on plates and serve with the minty yogurt and flatbreads or pitta bread, if you like.

A tangy South American sauce for steak, this makes a delicious Saturday night treat, especially served with chips/fries. A 2cm/¾in thick steak takes about 5 minutes for medium-rare if it was at room temperature before cooking and the pan is really hot. Leftover sauce will keep for a few days in the refrigerator to serve with grilled/broiled, roast or fried chicken or fish. You can also use it as a marinade or toss it into cooked vegetables.

Pan-fried Chimichurri Steak

MAKES 2 adult portions
PREPARATION TIME 10 minutes
COOKING TIME 5 minutes

FOR THE STEAKS
a drizzle of oil
2 good-quality steaks, whichever cut you prefer, such as rib-eye, rump, sirloin or fillet, left at room temperature for about 30 minutes before cooking
sea salt and freshly ground black pepper

FOR THE CHIMICHURRI SAUCE
1 tbsp chopped flat-leaf parsley leaves
1 tsp fresh oregano leaves
2 garlic cloves, roughly chopped
3 tbsp extra virgin olive oil
1 tbsp red wine vinegar
a pinch of dried chilli/hot pepper flakes

TO SERVE
½ recipe quantity Oven-baked Chips (see below) or shop-bought chips/fries
roasted vine tomatoes (optional)

1 To make the chimichurri sauce, put the parsley, oregano and garlic in a small food processor or blender and whizz until finely chopped, then stir in the extra virgin olive oil, red wine vinegar and chilli/hot pepper flakes. Season with salt and pepper and leave to one side until ready to serve.

2 To cook the steaks, put a griddle or large frying pan over a high heat and leave to become super-hot, then add a trickle of oil. If the steaks are at all wet, pat them dry with paper towels, then season generously with salt and pepper. As soon as the oil is smoking hot, put the steaks into the pan. Cook for about 1½ minutes, then flip over, cooking for a further minute or so, then flip over every minute until the steaks are cooked to your liking. If there is a thick piece of fat around the edge of the steak, use a pair of tongs to hold the steak vertically in the pan to brown the fat.

3 Remove the steaks from the pan and leave in a warm place to rest for at least 5 minutes. Serve the steaks with any resting juices poured over, and spoon some chimichurri sauce on top. Serve with oven-baked chips/fries and roasted vine tomatoes, if you like.

How to make
oven-baked chips, fries or wedges

Put a large, non-stick baking or roasting pan in the oven and preheat it to 200°C/400°F/gas 6. Cut **750g/1lb 10oz potatoes** or **sweet potatoes** into chip shapes or slim wedges, peeled or not, as you prefer. Toss in **3 tbsp olive oil** and transfer to the hot pan. Bake for 25–45 minutes (depending on the thickness of the potatoes), turning every 10 minutes or so until golden and cooked through. Once cooked, season with **salt** to your taste. For added flavour, toss **2 tsp dried spices** with the potatoes before cooking. My favourites are **paprika**, **mild chilli powder**, **garam masala**, **sumac**, **Cajun** or **Creole** seasoning. Choose flavours that complement the main dish. This makes enough for 4 adult portions.

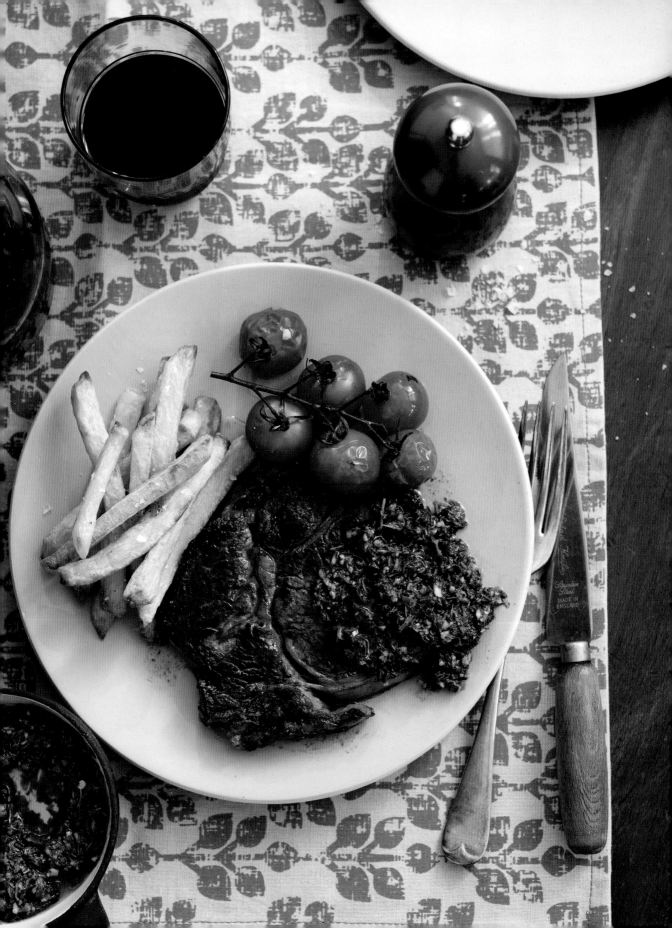

For an Asian twist on *moules-frîtes*, this makes a fabulous main-course dish served with some Oven-baked Chips (see page 148) or shop-bought chips/fries seasoned with sea salt and finely grated lime zest.

Fragrant Coconut and Chilli Mussels

MAKES 2 adult portions
PREPARATION TIME 15 minutes
COOKING TIME 15 minutes

1kg/2lb 4oz fresh mussels
1 tbsp sunflower oil
2 shallots, finely chopped
1 red chilli, deseeded and finely sliced
2cm/¾in piece of root ginger, peeled
  and finely chopped
1 lemongrass stalk, finely chopped
150ml/5fl oz/scant ⅔ cup white wine
150ml/5fl oz/scant ⅔ cup coconut cream
2 tsp Thai fish sauce
finely grated zest and juice of 1 lime
1 small handful of coriander/cilantro
  leaves, chopped

TO SERVE
½ recipe quantity Oven-baked Chips
  (see page 148) or shop-bought
  chips/fries
sea salt

1 Scrub the mussels thoroughly with a stiff brush under cold running water to remove all traces of grit, then remove any barnacles or other debris attached to the shells and pull off and discard any beards. Rinse again and discard any mussels that stay open.

2 Heat the oil in a wok or large saucepan over a medium heat, add the shallots, chilli, ginger and lemongrass and fry for 4–5 minutes until the shallots have softened but not coloured. Increase the heat to high, stir in the wine and bring to the boil. Carefully toss in the mussels, stir around, then cover the pan with a lid or, if you don't have one big enough, cover with a baking sheet. Cook for 5–6 minutes until the mussels have opened, shaking the pan a couple of times. Discard any that remain closed or will not open easily.

3 Stir in the coconut cream, fish sauce and lime juice and cook for 1 minute, stirring. Using a slotted spoon, lift the mussels out of the pan into bowls. Return the wok or pan to the heat and boil for a couple of minutes to reduce the sauce in quantity and thicken it slightly. Stir in the coriander/cilantro and pour over the mussels.

4 Sprinkle with the grated lime zest and serve with chips/fries seasoned lightly with sea salt.

It's Saturday night, the kids are all fast asleep (fingers crossed) and I'm reliably informed that mushrooms have considerable aphrodisiac qualities. I'll say no more …

Your Lucky Night Gnocchi

MAKES 2 adult portions
PREPARATION TIME 10 minutes, plus 20 minutes soaking
COOKING TIME 15 minutes

15g/½oz dried porcini, morel or mixed wild mushrooms
350–500g/12oz–1lb 2oz shop-bought gnocchi (depending on how hungry you are)
1 tbsp olive oil
40g/1½oz butter
100g/3½oz chestnut mushrooms, thinly sliced
2 garlic cloves, crushed
125ml/4fl oz/½ cup half-fat crème fraîche or sour cream
25g/1oz/¼ cup freshly grated Parmesan cheese
a squeeze of lemon juice
1 small handful of flat-leaf parsley leaves, chopped
sea salt and freshly ground black pepper

1 Cover the dried mushrooms with hot water and leave to soak for about 15–20 minutes.

2 Bring a pan of salted water to the boil, add the gnocchi and return to the boil. Cook for 2 minutes, then drain well.

3 Meanwhile, heat a large frying pan over a medium heat, add the olive oil and butter and heat until the butter is bubbling. Add the chestnut mushrooms and cook for 5–6 minutes until softened.

4 Drain the dried mushrooms, reserving the soaking liquid, and squeeze out any excess water. Add the mushrooms to the frying pan with the garlic and cook for a couple of minutes. Stir in the crème fraîche, about 100ml/3½fl oz/scant ½ cup of the mushroom liquid, the Parmesan, lemon juice and parsley. Season lightly with salt and pepper and cook until thoroughly hot but not quite boiling (or the crème fraîche may curdle).

5 Toss in the gnocchi and cook in the pan for a minute or so to soak up the flavours. Serve the gnocchi with a little extra mushroom liquid spooned over the top.

Unless you are entertaining, puddings tend to be the last thing on your mind. All you want to do is have a nice main course, then fall asleep halfway through a film. But this pud is so simple to make and so moreish, it might even give you the impetus to stay awake through the other half of that film. Why not try thinly sliced pears, peaches, plums, apricots or apple instead of the figs.

Fig Tartlets with Orange Mascarpone

MAKES 2 adult portions
PREPARATION TIME 15 minutes
COOKING TIME 15 minutes

FOR THE ORANGE MASCARPONE
100g/3½oz mascarpone
finely grated zest of ½ small orange
½ tsp vanilla extract
2 tbsp icing/confectioners' sugar, sifted
1 tbsp milk

FOR THE FIG TARTLETS
butter, for greasing
⅓ ready-rolled puff pastry sheet
2 tbsp apricot jam
2–3 ripe figs, very thinly sliced
1 egg yolk
1 tbsp milk
icing/confectioners' sugar, for dusting

1 Beat together all the orange mascarpone ingredients until you have a smooth cream. (You can prepare the mascarpone up to 24 hours in advance and keep it in the refrigerator.)

2 Preheat the oven to 200°C/400°F/gas 6 and lightly grease a large baking sheet with butter.

3 Cut the pastry into 2 heart shapes or circles about 10cm/4in in diameter using a sharp knife. Put onto the prepared baking sheet, and score a small border of about 1cm/½in around the edge of each one and prick the centre a couple of times with a fork.

4 Put 1 tbsp of the apricot jam in the centre of each piece of pastry. Arrange the figs in a circle on top of each piece of pastry. (The tartlets can be made a good few hours ahead of cooking and kept covered with cling film/plastic wrap in the refrigerator at this stage.) Mix together the egg yolk and milk to make an egg wash. Brush over the top of the figs and the pastry edges with the egg wash and then dust each one fairly generously with icing/confectioners' sugar. Bake for 15 minutes until the pastry is puffed up and golden around the edges.

5 Dust the tartlets with icing/confectioners' sugar and serve hot, warm or cool with a good spoonful of the orange mascarpone.

Leftovers for lunch
cheesy tomato pastries
Cut any remaining **puff pastry** into 2–4 rectangles and spread **a little Dijon mustard** or **tomato ketchup** onto one half of the surface. Scatter with a rubbery-type cheese, such as **grated Edam, Gouda, Gruyère, Emmental** or **Jarlsberg**, and add **1–2 slices of tomato**. Mix together **1 egg yolk** and **1 tbsp milk** to make an egg wash. Brush the edges of the pastry with the egg wash and fold over the other half of pastry, sealing the edges by pressing with the back of a fork. Put the pastries on a greased baking sheet, brush the top with a little more egg wash and scatter with more cheese. Bake in a preheated oven at 220°C/425°F/gas 7 for 10–12 minutes. Cool for a few minutes before serving.

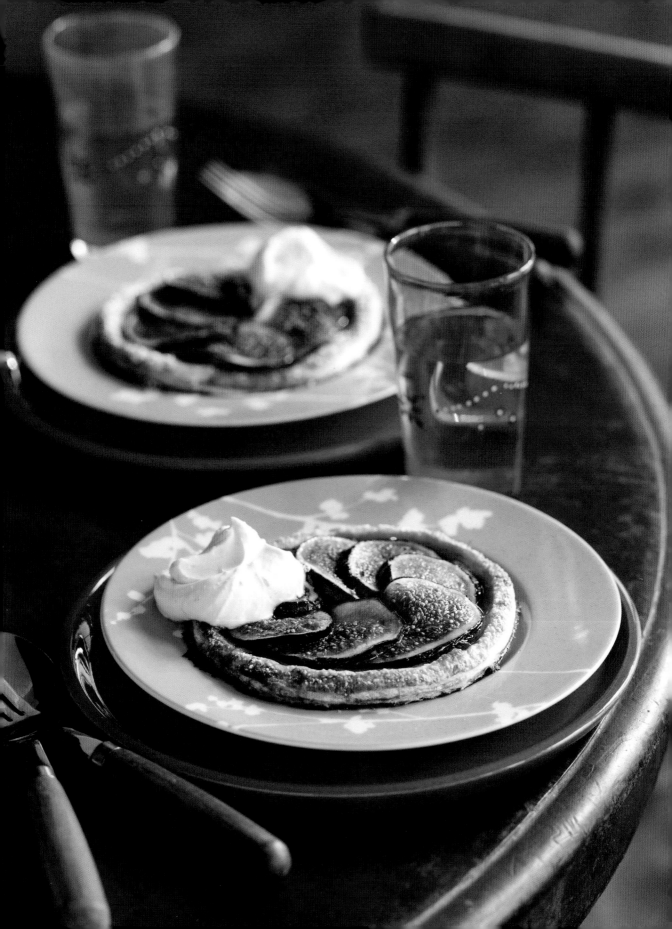

I love desserts that are simple yet look impressive – and here is one that ticks all the boxes. You can use other kinds of biscuits if you like. Ginger biscuits with lemon yogurt make a good combination.

Easy Yet Impressive Raspberry Cheesecake Pots

MAKES 2 adult portions
PREPARATION TIME 10 minutes, plus at least 30 minutes chilling

3 digestive biscuits/Graham crackers
1 tbsp butter, melted
125g/4½oz cream cheese
75ml/2½fl oz/scant ⅓ cup raspberry yogurt
2 tbsp icing/confectioners' sugar
finely grated zest of ½ lemon, plus 1 tsp grated lemon zest, to decorate
100g/3½oz/⅔ cup raspberries
2 tbsp shop-bought raspberry coulis or sauce

1 Put the digestive biscuits/Graham crackers in a food processor and blitz until they become fine crumbs. Alternatively, you can put the biscuits in a sandwich bag and crush with a rolling pin. Mix the crumbs with the melted butter and then press the mixture into the base of two glasses or dishes.

2 Mix together the cream cheese, yogurt, icing/confectioners' sugar and lemon zest until smooth. You may find a balloon whisk best for this. Mix the raspberries with the coulis or sauce. Make alternate layers of the raspberries and the cheesecake mixture on top of the cookie bases.

3 Put in the refrigerator to chill for at least 30 minutes. (The finished pots can be made a good couple of hours ahead and kept in the refrigerator.) Serve decorated with the 1 tsp grated lemon zest.

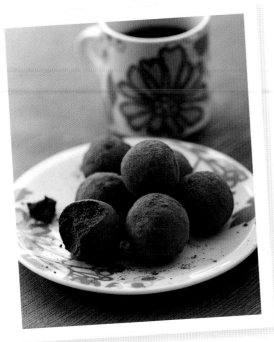

Leftovers for liqueur treats
boozy chocolate truffles

If you have opened a packet of digestive biscuits/Graham crackers especially for the cheesecake pots, the leftovers are ideal to make into these delicious chocolate truffles. Keep them simple for the kids or add some booze for an after-dinner treat for the grown-ups. Finely crush **8 digestive biscuits/Graham crackers**. Melt together **75g/2½oz dark chocolate, 70% cocoa solids, 1 tbsp golden/light corn syrup, 1 tbsp unsweetened cocoa powder** and **50g/1¾oz butter.** Add about **2 tbsp of your favourite liqueur** (such as brandy, whisky, orange liqueur, rum, coconut liqueur or whatever you like). Mix in the biscuits and shape into balls. Roll in a little unsweetened cocoa powder, then chill to set.

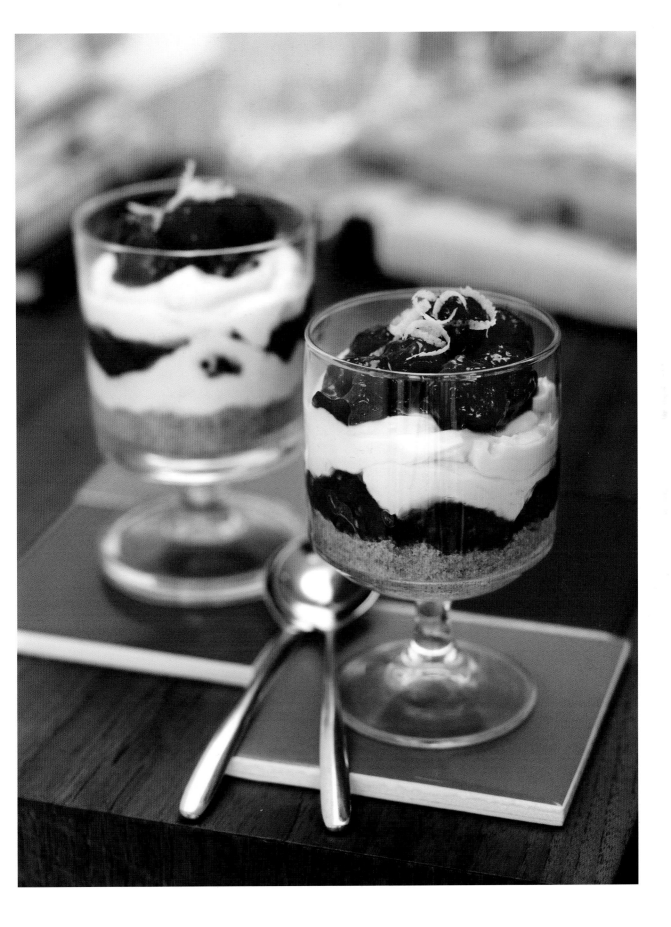

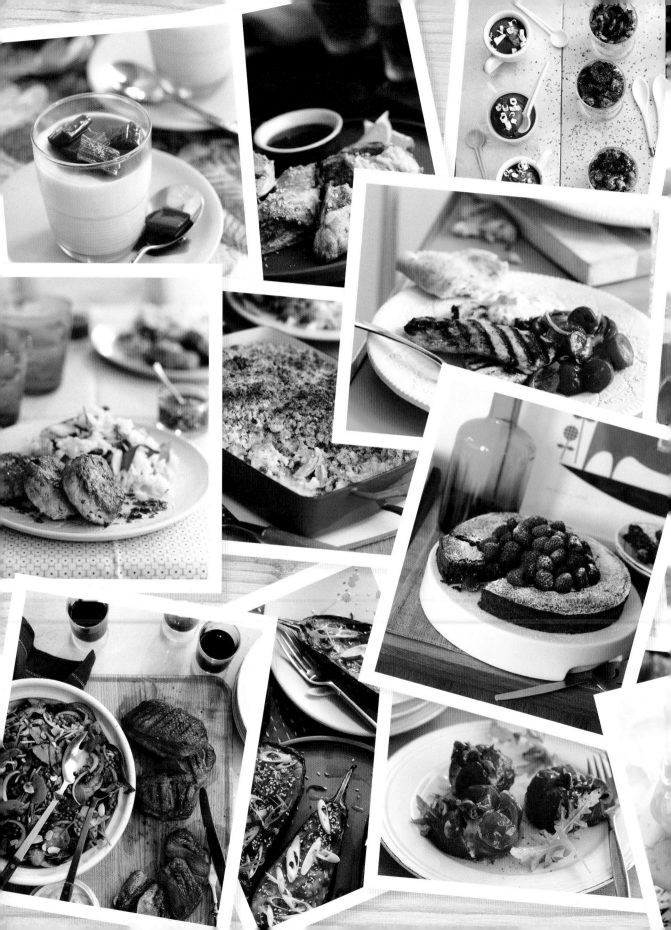

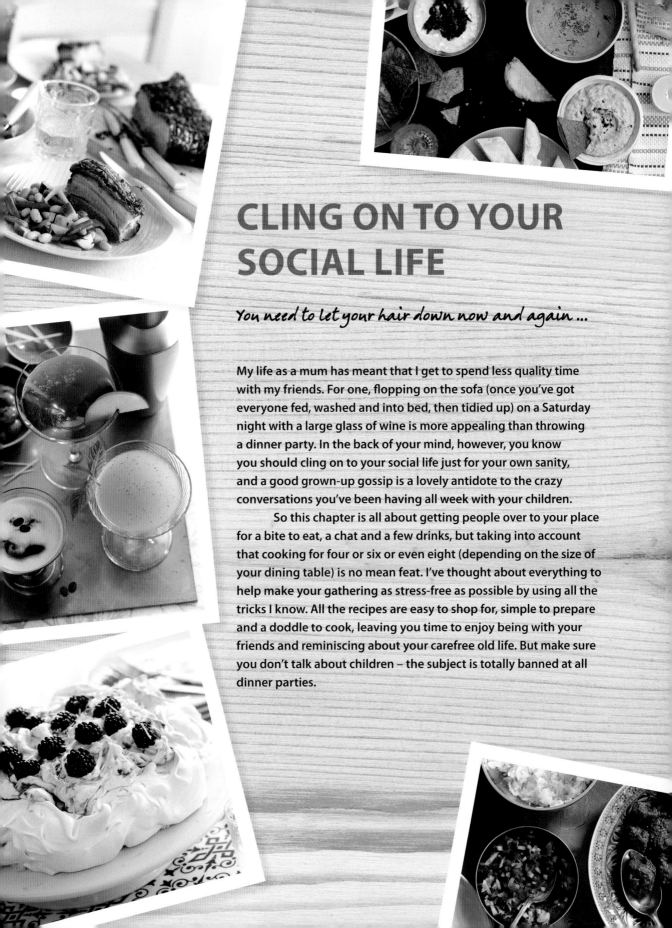

CLING ON TO YOUR SOCIAL LIFE

You need to let your hair down now and again ...

My life as a mum has meant that I get to spend less quality time with my friends. For one, flopping on the sofa (once you've got everyone fed, washed and into bed, then tidied up) on a Saturday night with a large glass of wine is more appealing than throwing a dinner party. In the back of your mind, however, you know you should cling on to your social life just for your own sanity, and a good grown-up gossip is a lovely antidote to the crazy conversations you've been having all week with your children.

So this chapter is all about getting people over to your place for a bite to eat, a chat and a few drinks, but taking into account that cooking for four or six or even eight (depending on the size of your dining table) is no mean feat. I've thought about everything to help make your gathering as stress-free as possible by using all the tricks I know. All the recipes are easy to shop for, simple to prepare and a doddle to cook, leaving you time to enjoy being with your friends and reminiscing about your carefree old life. But make sure you don't talk about children – the subject is totally banned at all dinner parties.

As a tasty alternative to a classic Peach Bellini, this sweet mango and fragrant lychee cocktail makes a lovely combination, but you don't have to stop here. Try some other types of soft fruit, such as raspberries or even a mixture of berries – in fact, go mad! Become famous for your fruity combos among your friends, open a Bellini bar, turn it into a franchise and become rich beyond your wildest dreams …

Mango and Lychee Bellini

MAKES 8 glasses
PREPARATION TIME 10 minutes

1 large ripe mango, pitted, peeled and
   roughly chopped
8 canned lychees, plus 2 tbsp of the
   lychee juice or syrup
1 bottle of chilled Prosecco, cava or
   Champagne

1 Put the mango and lychees in a blender with the juice and blend until you have a really smooth purée. (The purée can be made a couple of days in advance and kept in the refrigerator.)

2 Divide the purée into 8 Champagne flutes and pour in a little sparkling wine. Stir to mix, then slowly top up the glasses with the remaining sparkling wine.

How to make

berry purée

If you prefer your Bellini with berries, here's how to make the purée. Blend **200g/7oz fresh or frozen berries** to a smooth purée. Have a taste and if they seem quite sharp, add **a little sifted icing/confectioners' sugar** until they taste how you like them. Press the purée through a sieve/fine-mesh strainer/ fine-mesh strainer, leaving any pips and seeds behind. To make up the Bellini, half fill Champagne flutes with **chilled sparkling wine** or **Champagne**, then stir in **1 tbsp of the purée** and **1 tbsp berry liqueur**, such as crème de cassis (blackcurrant), chambord (raspberry), crème du muré (blackberry) or kirsch (cherry). Stir to mix and slowly top up with more sparkling wine. Any leftover purée can be kept in the refrigerator for a few days or stored in the freezer for up to 3 months.

Leftovers for an ice cream sauce

mango and lychee purée

It's well worth making extra purée so you have plenty more than you need. It's delicious **poured onto ice cream** to make a sundae, **stirred into whipped cream** for desserts or **mixed into yogurt**. I really like to **freeze it in ice-cube trays** so I can enjoy a cheeky little Mango and Lychee Bellini any time I fancy it.

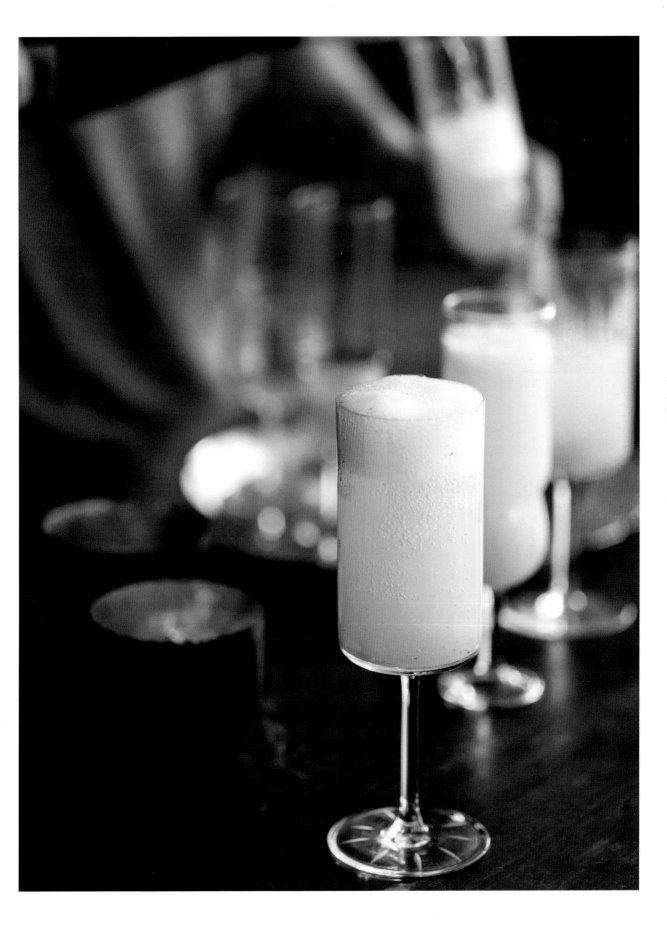

The traditional Moscow Mule is a combination of vodka, ginger beer and lime – so it has quite a kick. I started with the basic recipe and played around with it a bit in order to create my own version, with mint and angostura bitters. If vodka is not your spirit of choice, try one of the alternatives I've suggested, or try out some new ideas of your own – recipe testing cocktails doesn't count towards your weekly alcohol units (well that's my rule).

Travelling Mules

MAKES 2 glasses
PREPARATION TIME 5 minutes

FOR MOSCOW MULE
ice cubes
100ml/3½fl oz/scant ½ cup vodka
2 tbsp lime juice
250ml/9fl oz/1 cup chilled ginger beer
Angostura bitters
mint sprigs and thin slices of ginger,
   to serve

FOR TRAVELLING MULES
to ring the changes, swap the vodka
   for a different spirit:
FOR JAMAICAN MULE
dark, white or spiced rum
FOR MEXICAN MULE
tequila
FOR ENGLISH MULE
gin

1 Half fill two tall glasses with ice cubes. Divide the vodka and lime juice between the glasses and stir.

2 Top up with ginger beer, add a couple of shakes of Angostura bitters to each glass and stir again.

3 Decorate with mint sprigs and thin slices of ginger to serve.

A perfect drink to serve when it's chilly, you can even make it child or driver friendly by making it without the booze. Other options would be to make it with brandy, or a vanilla vodka would be nice.

Hot Apple Spice Punch

MAKES 8 large glasses
PREPARATION TIME 15 minutes

1.5l/52fl oz/6 cups apple juice
250ml/9fl oz/1 cup calvados (apple brandy)
4 cinnamon sticks
1 tsp whole cloves
1 tsp allspice berries
55g/2oz/¼ cup demerara sugar
peeled strips of orange zest from 2 oranges

1 Put all the ingredients in a saucepan over a medium-low heat. Making sure it doesn't boil, stir until the sugar has dissolved.

2 Continue to heat gently for about 10 minutes to allow all the flavours to infuse. Serve hot in heatproof glasses or cups.

Leftovers for a Gallic supper
pork chops with apple cream sauce

You can stir some **calvados** into **whipped cream** to serve with **apple or pear tarts**, **crumbles**, **pies** or **sponges**, or make this delicious pork dish. Cook **2 pork chops** in a frying pan over a medium-low heat for about 7–8 minutes on each side until cooked through, then leave to rest. Increase the heat to high, add **½ peeled, cored and finely diced apple** and **80ml/ 2½fl oz/⅓ cup calvados** and bubble for about 30 seconds, then add **100ml/3½fl oz/scant ½ cup double/heavy cream** and **1 tbsp chopped sage**. Bring to the boil and cook for 30 seconds, season lightly with **sea salt** and **freshly ground black pepper** and serve poured over the pork chops.

I love a martini to kick-start an evening and to welcome my friends to a fun night ahead. Apple, Elderflower and Cassis has turned into my signature Madhouse Martini – mainly due to the fact that I usually have all the ingredients and can shake one together in no time at all. Lemongrass, Ginger and Mint is tangy and aromatic, and ideal to serve before Asian cuisine. And to end an evening on a high, the Espresso Martini is an absolute must for coffee lovers.

Madhouse Martinis

EACH ONE MAKES 2 glasses
PREPARATION TIME 10 minutes each

APPLE, ELDERFLOWER AND CASSIS MARTINI

ice cubes
100ml/3½fl oz/scant ½ cup gin
100ml/3½fl oz/scant ½ cup apple juice
30ml/1fl oz/2 tbsp elderflower cordial
1 tbsp crème de cassis
thin slices of apple, to serve

1 Half fill a cocktail shaker with ice, then add the gin, apple juice, elderflower cordial and crème de cassis. Shake for a good 30 seconds.

2 Pour into two martini glasses and serve with thin slices of apple.

LEMONGRASS, GINGER AND MINT MARTINI

1 stalk of lemongrass, roughly chopped
about 15 mint leaves, plus extra to
   garnish
1½ balls stem ginger, roughly chopped
ice cubes
4 tbsp stem ginger syrup
125ml/4fl oz/½ cup vodka
juice of ½ lime

1 Put the lemongrass, mint leaves and stem ginger in a pestle and mortar, mini food processor or even a strong sandwich bag and bash or whizz to a rough paste. (This can be done well ahead of time and kept in the refrigerator until needed.) Transfer to a cocktail shaker half filled with ice, then add the ginger syrup, vodka and lime juice. Shake for a good 30 seconds.

2 Strain through a fine sieve/fine-mesh strainer or tea strainer into two martini glasses and serve with extra mint leaves.

ESPRESSO MARTINI

ice cubes
80ml/2½fl oz/⅓ cup freshly made
   espresso coffee
80ml/2½fl oz/⅓ cup vodka
80ml/2½fl oz/⅓ cup Kahlua or Tia Maria
   coffee liqueur
2 tbsp crème de cacao chocolate liqueur
   (optional)
a few whole coffee beans, to serve

1 Half fill a cocktail shaker with ice, then add the hot espresso, vodka, coffee liqueur and crème de cacao, if using. Shake for a good 30 seconds.

2 Pour into two martini glasses, add a couple of coffee beans and serve.

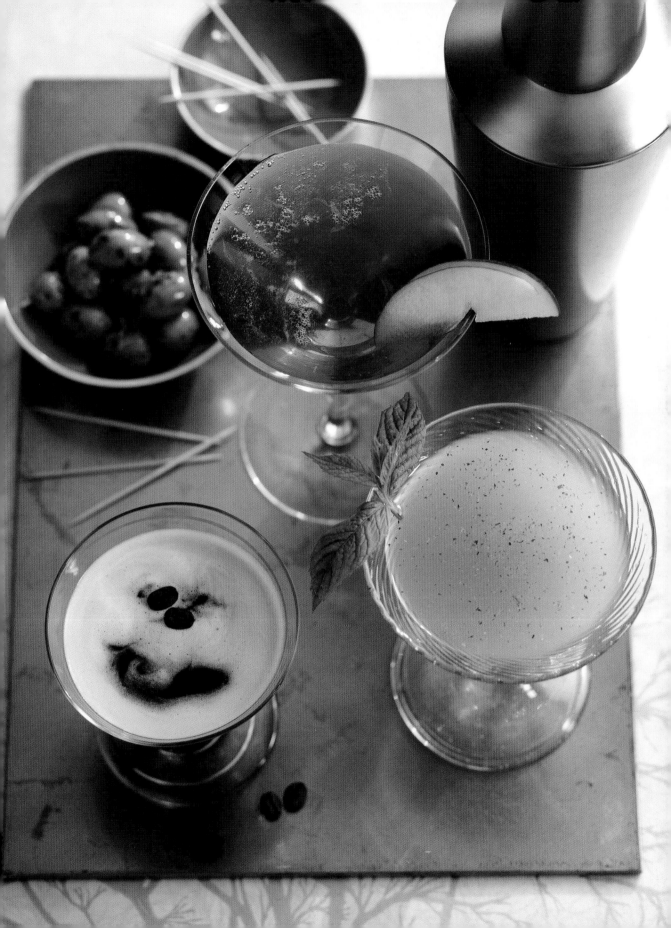

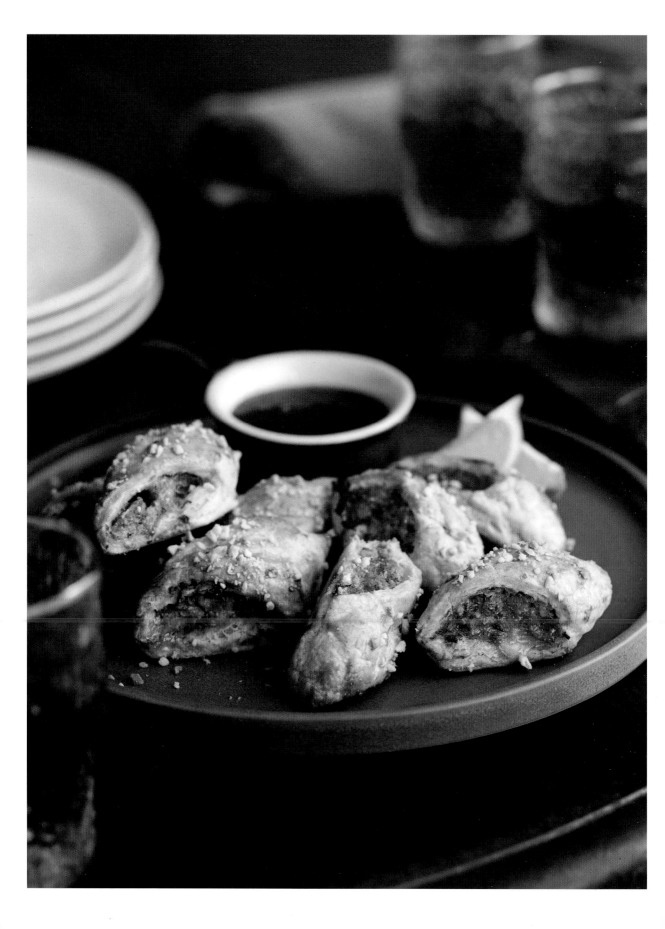

You can make these as spicy as you like (the spicier the better in my house so the kids won't eat them all before my guests arrive) but, whatever you do, make plenty, as they are very more-ish.

Thai Sausage and Peanut Rolls

MAKES about 30 rolls
PREPARATION TIME 25 minutes
COOKING TIME 25 minutes

oil, for greasing
50g/1¾oz/⅓ cup unsalted, skinned
  peanuts
250g/9oz sausage meat
1–2 tbsp Thai red curry paste
  (depending on how much spice you
  want)
1 large handful of coriander/cilantro
  leaves, roughly chopped
375g/13oz ready-rolled puff pastry
flour, for dusting
1 egg yolk
1 tbsp milk

TO SERVE
chilli dipping sauce
1 lime, cut into wedges

1 Preheat the oven to 190°C/375°F/gas 5 and grease a baking sheet.

2 Put the peanuts in a food processor and whizz until finely chopped. Remove one-third from the bowl and leave to one side. Add the sausage meat, Thai red curry paste and coriander/cilantro to the food processor bowl and whizz to combine.

3 Lay the pastry out flat on a lightly floured surface and cut into two long strips. Mix together the egg yolk and milk to make an egg wash, then brush the borders of the pastry with a little of the egg wash. Using wet hands to stop it sticking to you, divide the sausage meat in half and shape each piece into a long, thin sausage, the length of the pastry. Put one on top of each pastry strip, then fold over the pastry to seal in the sausage meat. Roll the whole thing over so the sealed edge is underneath. (The sausage rolls can now be kept in the refrigerator for 24 hours, lightly covered with cling film/plastic wrap, or they can even be frozen for up to 3 months and defrosted before cooking.)

4 Using a sharp knife, cut into bite-size sausage rolls, discarding the pastry ends, and score a couple of slits in the top of each one. Brush with the remaining egg wash and scatter over the reserved peanuts. Carefully lift onto the prepared baking sheet and bake for 20–25 minutes until cooked through and golden.

5 Serve warm with chilli dipping sauce and lime wedges. (If you make these ahead of time, they can be reheated in a low oven.)

Most supermarkets sell packets of pre-cooked unsweetened pancakes, which are ideal to use for this recipe. If you can't get hold of pancakes, flour tortillas make a good alternative. A can of crab meat is a good substitute for smoked salmon.

Smoked Salmon, Caper and Dill Pancake Rolls

MAKES about 20 mini rolls
PREPARATION TIME 20 minutes

200g/7oz cream cheese
1½ tbsp chopped dill
1 tbsp capers, finely chopped
grated zest and juice of ½ lemon
4 shop-bought pancakes or home-made
  Foolproof Pancakes (see page 86)
150g/5½oz thinly sliced smoked salmon
sea salt and freshly ground black pepper

1 Mix together the cream cheese, dill, capers, lemon zest and juice until creamy, then season lightly with salt and pepper.

2 Spread the mixture over the pancakes, then top with the smoked salmon. Roll each pancake tightly to form a long roll. (You can now wrap the rolls in cling film/plastic wrap and keep in the refrigerator until needed. This can be done a day ahead.)

3 Trim away the ends and cut into neat 2.5cm/1in slices. If any happen to unroll, stick cocktail sticks/toothpicks through them to secure. Serve straight away or keep covered in the refrigerator until ready to serve.

Leftovers for more-ish pancakes
savoury baked pancakes
Any leftover pancakes make a great meal for the kids. Fill them with **baked beans**, **bolognese sauce**, **ratatouille** or **fish pie filling**. Roll them up and put them in an ovenproof dish, scatter with **grated cheese** and bake in a preheated oven at 200°C/400°F/gas 6 for about 10 minutes until golden and bubbling.

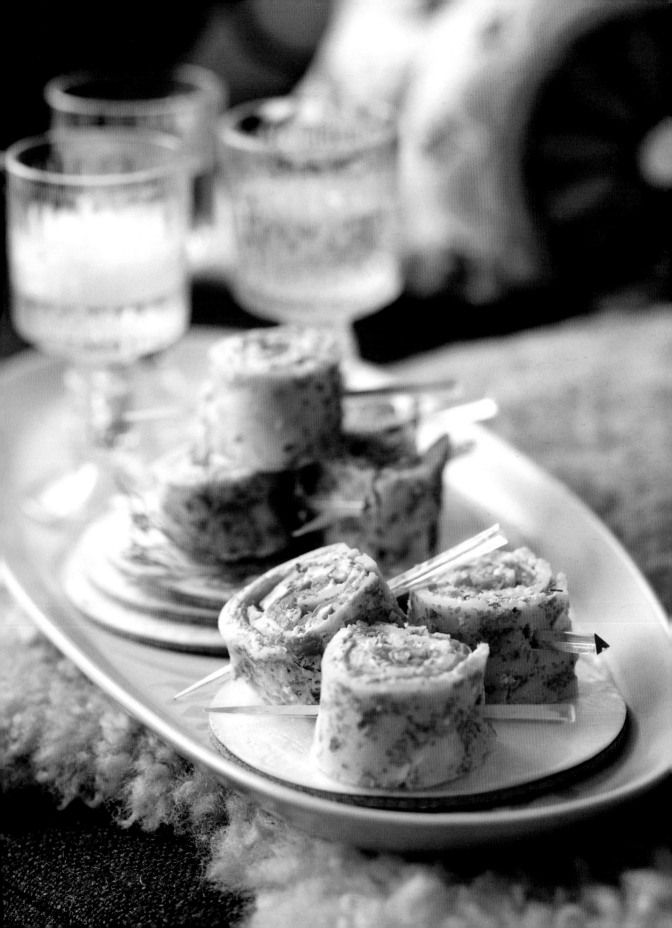

Of course, there's nothing to stop you using Beluga caviar instead of the cheaper version if you like! Ready-made blinis make the recipe even quicker and easier but it's very satisfying to make your own, so why not have a go with my recipe below.

Crab and Avocado Blinis

MAKES 12–16 blinis
PREPARATION TIME 15 minutes
COOKING TIME 10 minutes if cooking your own blinis

12–16 shop-bought mini or cocktail blinis or ½ recipe quantity Cocktail Blinis (below)
1 ripe avocado, halved and pitted
juice of ½ lemon
1 tbsp olive oil
a splash of Tabasco sauce
100g/3½oz fresh white crab meat
2–3 tbsp mayonnaise or seafood sauce
sea salt and freshly ground black pepper

TO SERVE
1–2 tsp lumpfish caviar (optional)
a few chives

1 If you are using shop-bought blinis, warm them according to the packet instructions. This will make them lighter in texture than if you used them straight from the packet. If you are making your own, follow the instructions below.

2 Scoop the flesh out of the avocado and mash with the back of a fork, then mix in a good squeeze of lemon juice, the oil and Tabasco and season lightly with salt and pepper.

3 In a separate bowl, mix together the crab meat, mayonnaise and a squeeze of lemon juice. Season with salt and pepper, if needed. Spoon the avocado mixture on top of the blinis, then top with some crab. Top each one with lumpfish caviar, if you like, and a small piece of chive.

4 Cover and keep in the refrigerator until you are ready to serve.

How to make
cocktail blinis

To make about 24 blinis, beat together **85g/3oz/⅔ cup buckwheat flour** with **1 tsp baking powder**, **1 lightly beaten egg** and **125ml/4fl oz/½ cup milk** and **a pinch of salt**. Heat **a drop of oil** in a frying pan over a medium heat until hot, then drop in spoonfuls of the batter and fry for a minute or so on each side until pale golden. Once cooked, they freeze really well.

These are so easy to put together and make a colourful plate of nibbles to entice your guests. For a slightly sweeter version, try spreading the pastry with a spoonful of cranberry sauce and some chunks of Brie.

Cherry Tomato and Feta Pastry Squares

MAKES about 30 squares
PREPARATION TIME 15 minutes
COOKING TIME 15 minutes

200g/7oz ready-rolled puff pastry
olive oil, for brushing
150g/5½oz feta cheese, crumbled
15 cherry tomatoes, halved
15 black olives, pitted and halved
sea salt and freshly ground black pepper

1 Preheat the oven to 200°C/400°F/gas 6 and line a baking sheet with baking paper.

2 Cut the pastry into 2.5cm/1in squares and put on the prepared baking sheet. Prick each square a few times with a fork. Brush over the pastry with olive oil, then top with crumbled feta. Put a tomato half and black olive on each one, then season lightly with salt and pepper. (They can be prepared up to this stage the day before required and kept in the refrigerator, loosely covered with cling film/plastic wrap.)

3 Bake for 15 minutes until golden. Serve warm or at room temperature.

Leftovers for mini pies
savoury or sweet pastry puffs

Get the kids involved in using up the leftover pastry. Use mini cutters to cut out pastry shapes and put them on a greased baking sheet lined with baking paper. Mix **1 egg yolk** with **1 tbsp milk** to make an egg wash and brush over the surface of the pastry. For a savoury version, top each one with **finely grated Parmesan cheese**, **Gruyère cheese**, **poppy seeds** or **sesame seeds**. For sweet pastry puffs, generously sprinkle over **caster/superfine sugar** or a **flavoured sugar**, such as vanilla sugar or cinnamon sugar. Bake in a preheated oven at 200°C/400°F/gas 6 for 5–8 minutes until puffed up and golden, then serve.

You can whizz together these delicious dips in minutes to serve with tortilla chips, crisps, breadsticks, pitta bread, carrot, cucumber, celery, peppers, radishes – or whatever you like. They can all be made a day in advance and stored in the refrigerator, but take them out 30 minutes before serving to get the most out of their flavours.

Quick Dips

EACH ONE MAKES 4–6 adult dip portions
PREPARATION TIME 5 minutes each

ARTICHOKE, ROCKET AND PARMESAN DIP

280g/10oz jar artichokes in oil
50g/1¾oz rocket/arugula leaves
50g/1¾oz/⅔ cup freshly grated Parmesan cheese
juice of ½ lemon
2 tbsp extra virgin olive oil
sea salt and freshly ground black pepper

1 Drain half of the oil from the artichokes and put the remaining oil with the artichokes in a food processor along with the rocket/arugula leaves, Parmesan, lemon juice and extra virgin olive oil. Season lightly with salt and pepper and whizz to a paste. Spoon into a serving bowl and chill in the refrigerator.

2 When ready, give the dip a little stir before serving.

CARAMELIZED ONION AND DOLCELATTE DIP

150g/5½oz dolcelatte cheese
150ml/5fl oz/scant ⅔ cup half-fat crème fraîche or sour cream
1 tbsp lemon juice
freshly ground black pepper
3 tbsp bottled caramelized onions

1 Whizz together the dolcelatte, crème fraîche, lemon juice and plenty of freshly ground black pepper in a food processor until smooth. You shouldn't need salt as the cheese is naturally salty, but add some if you think it needs it.

2 Spoon into a serving bowl and spoon the onions on top. Use the handle of a teaspoon to lightly swirl into the top of the cream cheese, and serve.

CREAMY MUSTARD AND SPRING ONION DIP

200ml/7fl oz/scant 1 cup half-fat crème fraîche or sour cream
1 tbsp Dijon mustard
2 tsp clear honey
4 spring onions/scallions, very finely chopped
sea salt

1 Simply mix everything together, spoon into a dish and serve.

BEETROOT AND SOUR CREAM DIP

200g/7oz cooked beetroot (not in
  vinegar)
100ml/3½fl oz/scant ½ cup sour cream
150ml/5fl oz/scant ⅔ cup mayonnaise
1 tbsp chopped chives
sea salt and freshly ground black pepper

1 Whizz the beetroot, sour cream, mayonnaise, salt and pepper in a food processor until smooth and a fabulous pink colour.

2 Spoon into a serving bowl and serve sprinkled with the chives.

SPICY WHITE BEAN AND RED PEPPER DIP

240g/8½oz canned white beans, either
  cannellini or butter beans, drained
2 bottled or canned roasted red peppers
50g/1¾oz/½ cup ground almonds
2 garlic cloves, crushed
juice of ½ lemon
½ tsp dried chilli/hot pepper flakes, plus
  extra for sprinkling
3 tbsp extra virgin olive oil, plus extra for
  drizzling
sea salt and freshly ground black pepper

1 Put all the ingredients in a food processor and whizz until smooth. Have a taste and add any extra seasoning, chilli/hot pepper flakes, lemon juice or extra virgin olive oil, depending on your personal preference.

2 Spoon into a serving bowl, add a drizzle of extra virgin olive oil and a sprinkling of chilli/hot pepper flakes, and serve.

PEA, GOATS' CHEESE AND MINT DIP

300g/10½oz/2 cups frozen peas,
  defrosted
150g/5½oz soft goats' cheese
1 large handful of mint leaves, plus extra
  for sprinkling
1 garlic clove, crushed
finely grated zest of 1 lemon
juice of ½ lemon, plus extra for
  sprinkling
2 tbsp extra virgin olive oil
sea salt and freshly ground black pepper

1 Whizz together the peas, goats' cheese, mint leaves, garlic, lemon zest and extra virgin olive oil in a food processor until you have a relatively smooth consistency. Add lemon juice and salt and pepper to taste.

2 Spoon into a serving bowl, add a sprinkling of extra mint leaves and/or lemon juice to serve.

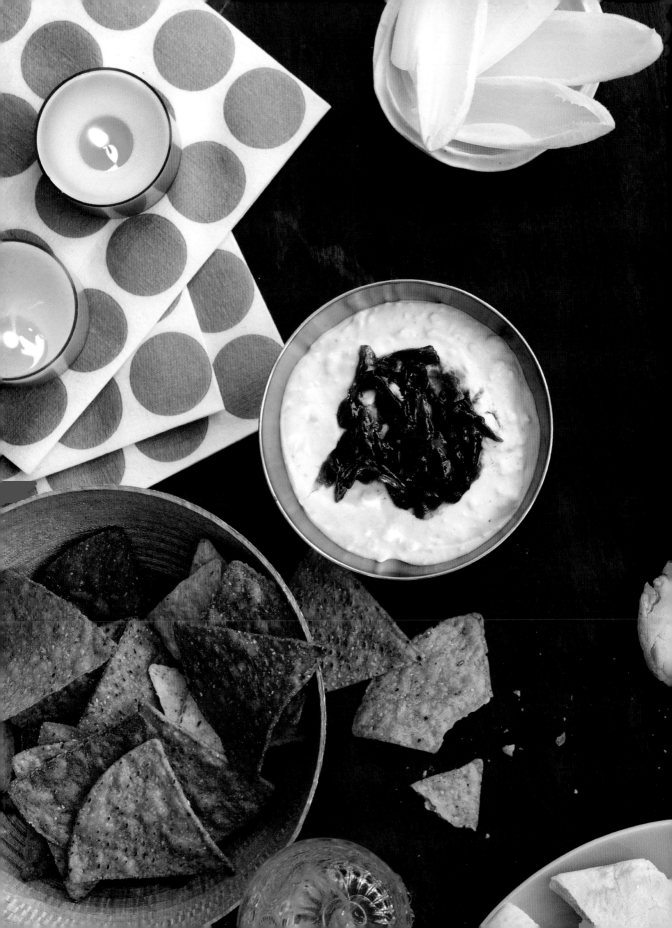

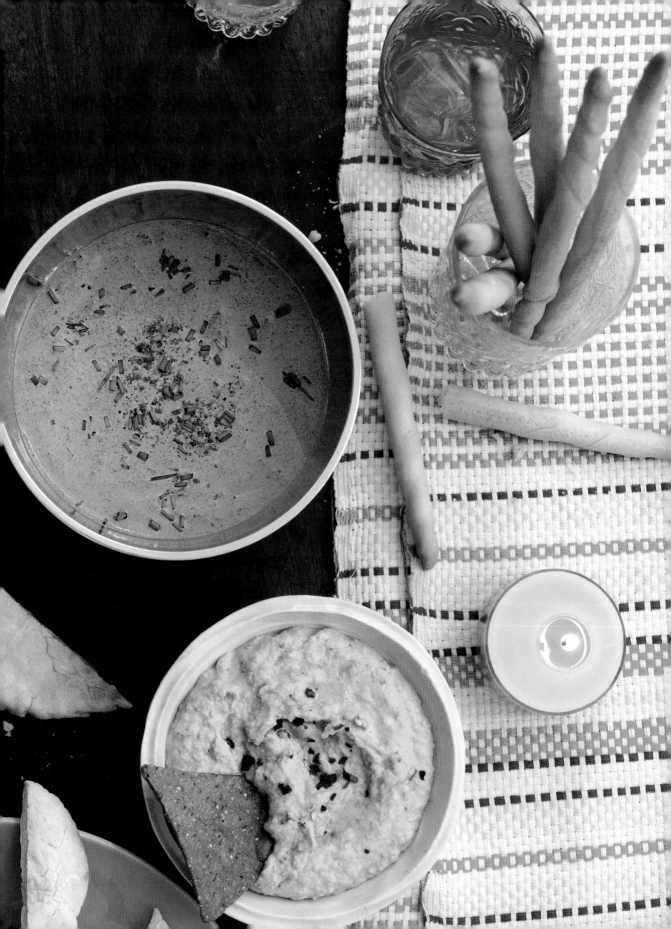

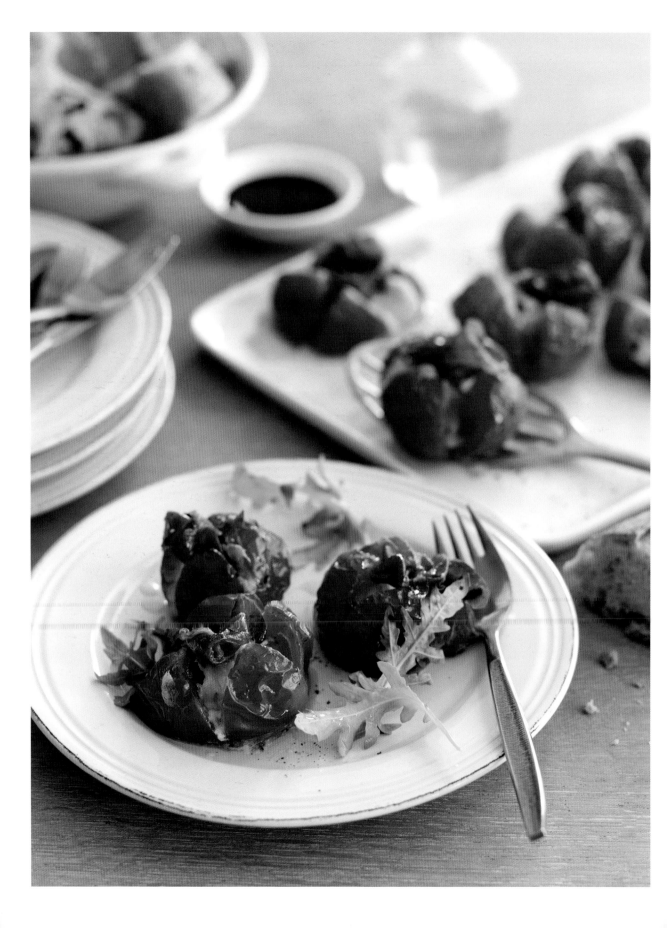

A few rocket/arugula leaves and some slices of fresh focaccia or ciabatta are perfect with this delicious starter, whether you serve it warm or cold. For best results, make sure your tomatoes are really ripe and juicy.

Mozzarella and Parma Baked Tomatoes

MAKES 4 adult portions
PREPARATION TIME 15 minutes
COOKING TIME 20 minutes

12 juicy, ripe tomatoes (roughly the size of golf balls)
125g/4½oz buffalo mozzarella, cut into 12 pieces
2 oregano sprigs
4 slices of Parma ham, each torn into 3 pieces
about 2 tbsp extra virgin olive oil
sea salt and freshly ground black pepper

TO SERVE
rocket/arugula leaves
fresh Italian bread
olive oil
balsamic vinegar

1 Preheat the oven to 180°C/350°F/gas 4 and line a baking sheet with baking paper or kitchen foil.

2 Cut a cross on the top of each tomato, cutting halfway down, then put them on the prepared baking sheet. Squeeze them very lightly to open the tomatoes up slightly, then season with salt and pepper. Gently press a piece of mozzarella into each tomato, followed by a couple of oregano leaves and a piece of Parma ham. Don't worry if it doesn't all fit in properly, as once they are in the oven the cheese will melt and the ham will fall into place. (If you are serving the tomatoes warm, they can be prepared up to this stage a couple of hours before going into the oven.)

3 Drizzle over the extra virgin olive oil, then bake for 15–20 minutes until the cheese is melted and the Parma ham is becoming golden.

4 Serve on individual plates or on a serving plate to share, with some peppery rocket/arugula leaves, fresh Italian bread and some olive oil and balsamic vinegar for dipping.

This is such an easy starter to prepare and the results are really impressive. Smoked mackerel has a delicious, rich flavour and texture that is perfectly complemented by the sweet and sour beetroot relish. If you have some beetroot left over from making this relish, why not try the Beetroot and Sour Cream Dip on page 171.

Smoked Mackerel and Horseradish Pâté with Beetroot Relish

MAKES 4 adult portions
PREPARATION TIME 20 minutes

**FOR THE SMOKED MACKEREL AND
   HORSERADISH PÂTÉ**
250g/9oz skinless smoked mackerel
   fillets
100ml/3½fl oz/scant ½ cup crème
   fraîche or sour cream
150g/5½oz cream cheese
1 tbsp hot horseradish sauce
2 tsp lemon juice
sea salt and freshly ground black pepper
toast, crispbread or bruschetta, to serve

FOR THE BEETROOT RELISH
125g/4½oz cooked beetroot, finely
   diced
2 tbsp shop-bought caramelized onions
a splash of balsamic vinegar
1 tbsp finely chopped flat-leaf parsley
   or thyme leaves

1 Flake the mackerel into a food processor, removing any bones that you might come across. Add the crème fraîche, cream cheese, horseradish, lemon juice and plenty of black pepper. Blend the pâté until smooth. Spoon into four individual dishes, cover and put in the refrigerator.

2 To make the relish, mix all the ingredients together in a bowl and season with a little salt and pepper. (Both the pâté and the relish can be prepared a day in advance and kept cold in the refrigerator.)

3 Serve the pâté with the relish and toast.

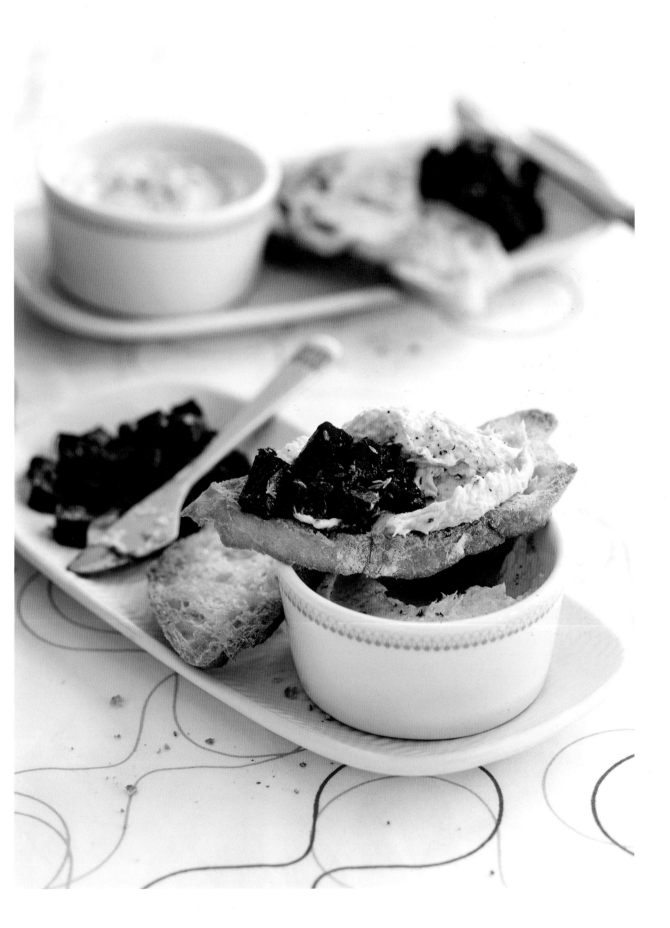

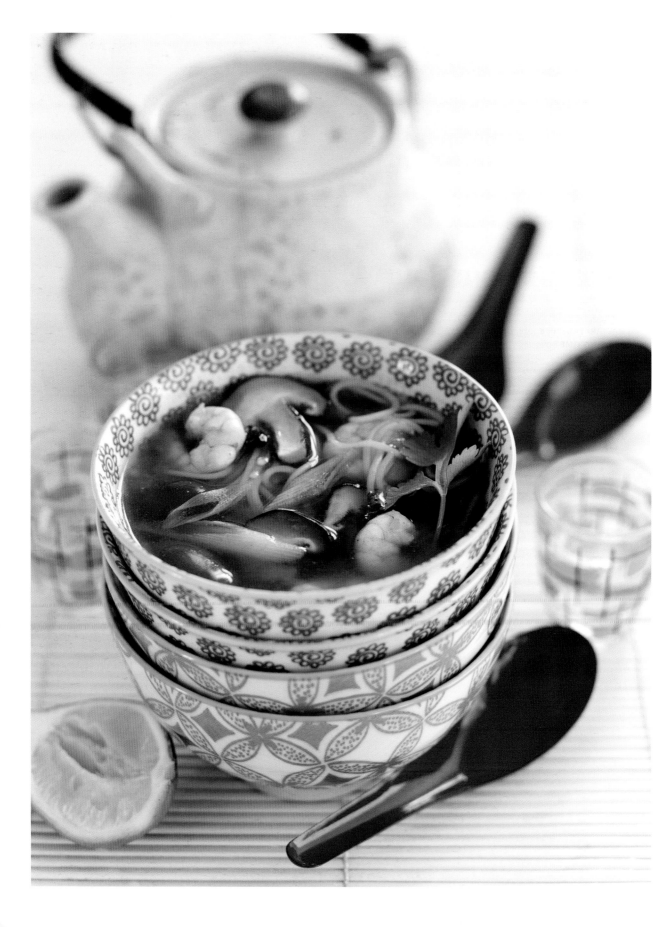

This light and flavoursome soup really has the wow factor – but the wonderful reality is that it's amazingly easy to make. If you fancy a change from prawns/shrimp, try using sliced chicken or tofu instead.

Hot and Sour Soup with Prawns

MAKES 4 adult portions
PREPARATION TIME 10 minutes
COOKING TIME 8 minutes

200g/7oz raw, peeled tiger prawns/
   jumbo shrimp
½ tsp sea salt
1½ tsp caster/superfine sugar
100g/3½oz vermicelli rice noodles
1l/35fl oz/4 cups vegetable stock
2 lemongrass stalks
2 tbsp Thai fish sauce
¼ tsp chilli paste
100g/3½oz shiitake mushrooms, thinly
   sliced
100g/3½oz baby plum tomatoes, halved
4 spring onions/scallions, finely sliced
juice of 1½ limes
3 fresh or dried kaffir lime leaves, torn
   into pieces
a few coriander/cilantro leaves, for
   sprinkling

1 Put the prawns/shrimp in a small bowl and stir in the salt and ½ tsp of the sugar. This will really bring out their flavour. Break the noodles into about 5cm/2in long pieces and soak them in hot water for a couple of minutes to soften, then drain. (You can get all the ingredients ready and prepare the recipe to this point, then put it in the refrigerator so you can do the last-minute cooking just before serving.)

2 Meanwhile, heat the stock in a wok or large saucepan over a medium heat. Bash the ends of the lemongrass to help release their delicious flavour, then add to the pan with the fish sauce, chilli paste and remaining sugar. Bring to the boil, then reduce the heat to low and leave to simmer for 5 minutes.

3 Drain the noodles and add to the wok along with the prawns/shrimp, shiitake mushrooms, tomatoes, spring onions/scallions, lime juice and kaffir lime leaves. Simmer for about 5 minutes until the prawns/shrimp are cooked through (they will have turned pink). Have a taste. If the soup could do with being slightly more spicy, add a little more chilli paste; if it's a little too hot, add some sugar and a squeeze of lime.

4 Serve sprinkled with a few coriander/cilantro leaves.

As always with chillis, taste and adjust the spiciness to suit what you like best. This is a great way to use up bread that's not super-fresh, or you can make the dish look much more sophisticated by using a fancy bread. The addition of sumac gives a distinctive tang but you can use a squeeze of lemon if you don't have any.

Crab and Chilli Toasts

MAKES 4 adult portions
PREPARATION TIME 15 minutes
COOKING TIME 5 minutes

200g/7oz fresh white crab meat
finely grated zest of 1 lemon
1 tsp sumac or crushed fennel seeds
2 tbsp chopped flat-leaf parsley leaves
2 tbsp extra virgin olive oil, plus extra
  for drizzling
½–1 red chilli, deseeded and finely
  chopped
4–8 slices of ciabatta or sourdough
  (depending on the size)
sea salt and freshly ground black pepper
watercress or rocket/arugula leaves,
  to serve

1 Put the white crab meat in a bowl and break up any chunks with your fingers or a fork. Add the lemon zest, sumac, parsley and extra virgin olive oil, and season lightly with salt and pepper. (The crab mixture can be made quite a few hours before you need it, covered and kept cold in the refrigerator.)

2 Drizzle the bread with some extra virgin olive oil, then lightly toast. If the slices are particularly large, cut them in half. Spoon the crab mixture onto the toasts and serve with a little watercress or rocket/arugula.

Leftovers for lemon-spiced veggies
sauté potatoes with sumac and thyme
An open jar of sumac can be used in a variety of ways but one that creates a real wow factor is to fry slices of leftover boiled potatoes in a combination of **olive oil** and **butter** until they are becoming golden and crispy. Add a good sprinkling of **sumac** and some **thyme leaves**. Continue to fry for a few more minutes before seasoning with **sea salt** and **freshly ground black pepper**. Serve with **fish**, **chicken** or simply topped with **a fried egg**.

Serve this delicious dish hot or chilled, depending on the weather. It's always a great favourite with the kids – they love the sweet flavour from the peas and the creamy texture – so it is well worth making more than you need and freezing any extra for a later date.

Pea and Watercress Soup with Tomato and Mint Salsa

MAKES 4 adult portions
PREPARATION TIME 15 minutes
COOKING TIME 10 minutes

FOR THE PEA AND WATERCRESS SOUP
2 tbsp olive oil
1 leek, sliced
800ml/28fl oz/scant 3½ cups chicken
   or vegetable stock
540g/1lb 3oz/3½ cups frozen peas
100g/3½oz watercress
100g/3½oz cream cheese
sea salt and freshly ground black pepper

FOR THE TOMATO AND MINT SALSA
4 ripe tomatoes, deseeded and diced
4 spring onions/scallions, chopped
1 handful of mint leaves, chopped
1 tbsp extra virgin olive oil
a small squeeze of lemon juice

1 Heat the oil in a saucepan over a low heat, add the leek and fry for about 5 minutes until it has softened but not coloured. Add the stock and bring to the boil, then add the peas and watercress. Return to the boil and cook for 3 minutes. Stir in the cream cheese and season with salt and pepper.

2 Blitz the soup in a food processor or blender, or by using a hand blender, until it is smooth. Check for seasoning and add extra if needed. (Prepare the soup up to a day in advance up to this stage, cool and keep chilled until you are ready to finish and serve.)

3 To make the salsa, mix together all the salsa ingredients and season with salt and pepper.

4 Serve the soup hot or cold, with the tomato salsa spooned over the top.

A lovely combination of flavours that make a light and tasty starter. If you have room to grow a few herbs in the garden, that's great as you'll always have supplies to hand. If not, keep a few growing in pots on the windowsill if you can.

Roast Mushroom Brioche with Goats' Cheese

MAKES 4 adult portions
PREPARATION TIME 15 minutes
COOKING TIME 20 minutes

75g/2½oz butter, at room temperature
2 tbsp chopped oregano leaves or
   1 tbsp chopped thyme leaves, plus
   extra leaves for sprinkling
2 plump garlic cloves, crushed
finely grated zest of ½ lemon
1 brioche loaf
4 large, flat white or chestnut/cremini
   mushrooms (about 8cm/5in diameter)
150g/5½oz mild soft goats' cheese
olive oil, for drizzling
sea salt and freshly ground black pepper

1 Preheat the oven to 200°C/400°F/gas 6 and line a baking sheet with baking paper.

2 Mix together the butter, oregano, garlic, lemon zest, salt and pepper.

3 Cut 4 slices of brioche about 3cm/1¼in thick. Spread half the herb butter onto one side of each piece of brioche. Top each one with a mushroom, stalk-side up, then spread the remaining butter over the mushrooms. (The mushroom brioche can be prepared to this stage a good few hours before they are needed. Cover with cling film/plastic wrap and keep in a cool place.)

4 Put the mushroom brioche on the prepared baking sheet and bake for 15–20 minutes until the mushrooms are tender and the brioche is a lovely golden brown.

5 Top each mushroom with a spoonful of goats' cheese, drizzle with olive oil and add a twist of black pepper, then sprinkle with oregano or thyme leaves and serve.

Leftovers for breakfast
hot jam brioche sandwich
For a comforting breakfast treat, sandwich a **couple of slices of brioche** together with **1 tbsp jam** or **marmalade**. Beat **1 egg** with **2 tsp sugar** (plain, vanilla or cinnamon) and soak the brioche in the egg until all the egg is absorbed. Fry in **melted butter** for 1–2 minutes on each side until golden. Sprinkle with **sugar** and enjoy.

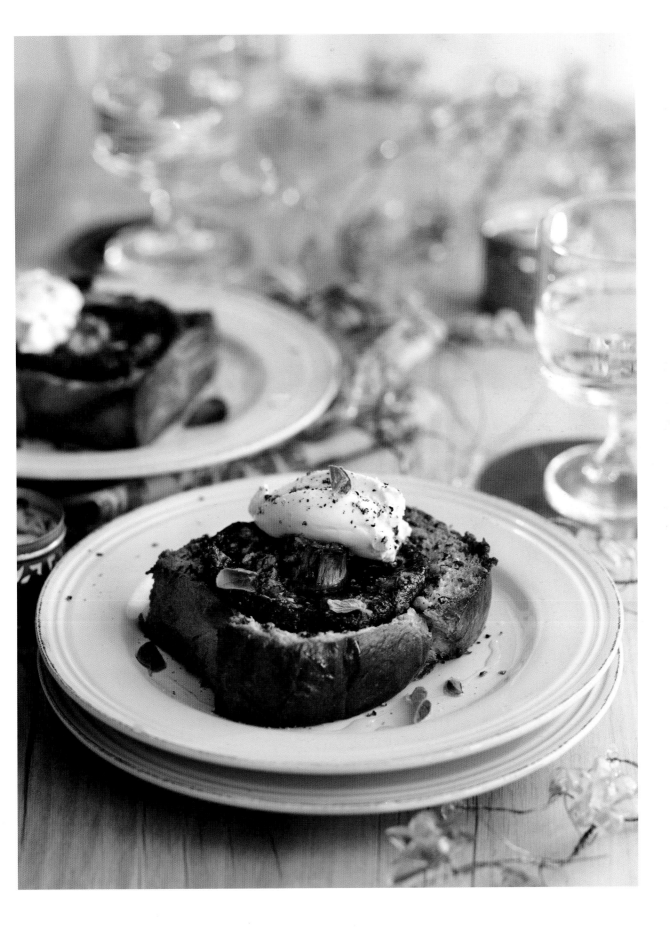

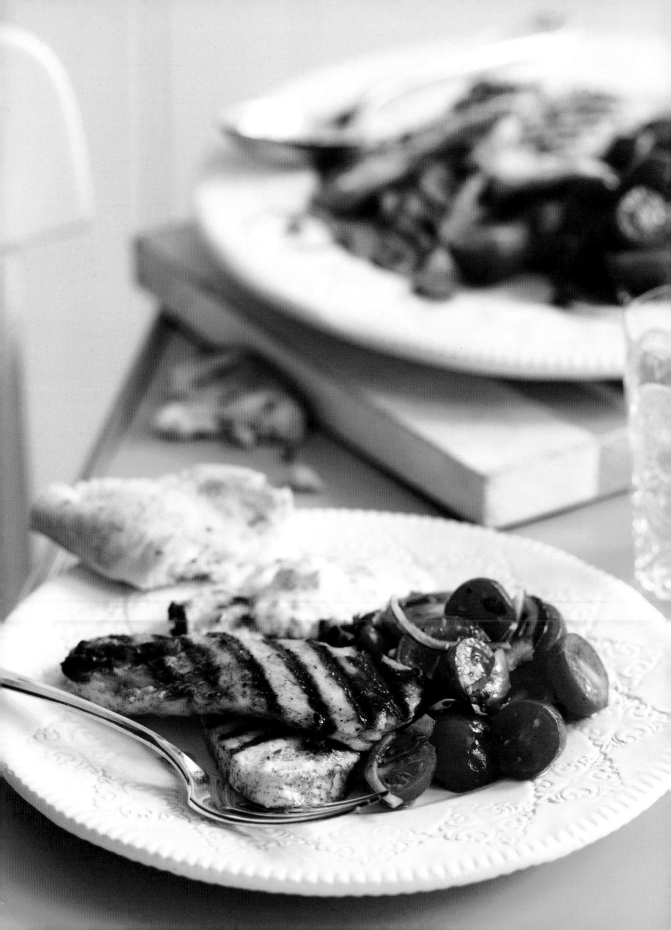

Halloumi cheese originally comes from Cyprus and is a firm cheese with a strong, salty flavour that is more than a match for the spices – in fact, you could say it's a match made in heaven!

Spicy Halloumi with Tomato and Coriander Salad

MAKES 4 adult portions
PREPARATION TIME 15 minutes, plus
 2 hours marinating
COOKING TIME 8 minutes

FOR THE SPICY HALLOUMI
375g/13oz halloumi cheese, cut into
 1cm/½in slices
2 tbsp olive oil
2 tsp garam masala
½ tsp chilli powder
a squeeze of lemon juice

**FOR THE TOMATO AND CORIANDER
 SALAD**
350g/12oz cherry tomatoes, halved
½ red onion, finely sliced
2 tbsp extra virgin olive oil
1 tbsp lemon juice
1 handful of coriander/cilantro leaves,
 chopped
sea salt and freshly ground black pepper

TO SERVE
4 tbsp plain yogurt or Cucumber Raita
 (see page 25) (optional)
warmed mini naan bread (optional)

1 Put the halloumi cheese in a non-metallic bowl or sandwich bag. Mix together the olive oil, garam masala, chilli powder and lemon juice. Pour over the halloumi and gently turn the cheese so it is coated in the spiced oil. Cover and leave to marinate in the refrigerator for 2 hours to absorb the flavours. (Ideally, the halloumi needs a couple of hours in the spiced oil, but you can leave it in the refrigerator all day if that's more convenient.)

2 Meanwhile, to make the salad, toss together the tomatoes, onion, extra virgin olive oil, lemon juice and coriander/cilantro. Season lightly with salt and pepper.

3 To cook the halloumi, heat a large frying pan or griddle over a medium-high heat, add the halloumi and fry for a couple of minutes on each side until golden. You may need to do this in batches; if so, put the hot halloumi onto a plate and keep warm by covering loosely with foil while you cook the remainder.

4 Spoon the halloumi on top of the salad and serve with the yogurt or raita and naan bread, if you like.

Leftovers for an Indian-style lunch
mini naan 'pizza'
If you plan to serve mini naan bread with this starter, grab an extra packet and make some quick Indian-inspired pizzas for the kids. Mix **1 tbsp mild curry paste** and **1 tbsp mango chutney** into **200g/7oz/scant 1 cup canned chopped tomatoes**. Spread over the top of **2 or 4 naan bread** (depending on their actual size). Top with **crumbled feta**, and a sprinkling each of defrosted **frozen peas** and **chopped spring onion/scallion**. Drizzle with **a little olive oil** and bake in a preheated oven at 220°C/425°F/gas 7 for about 10 minutes.

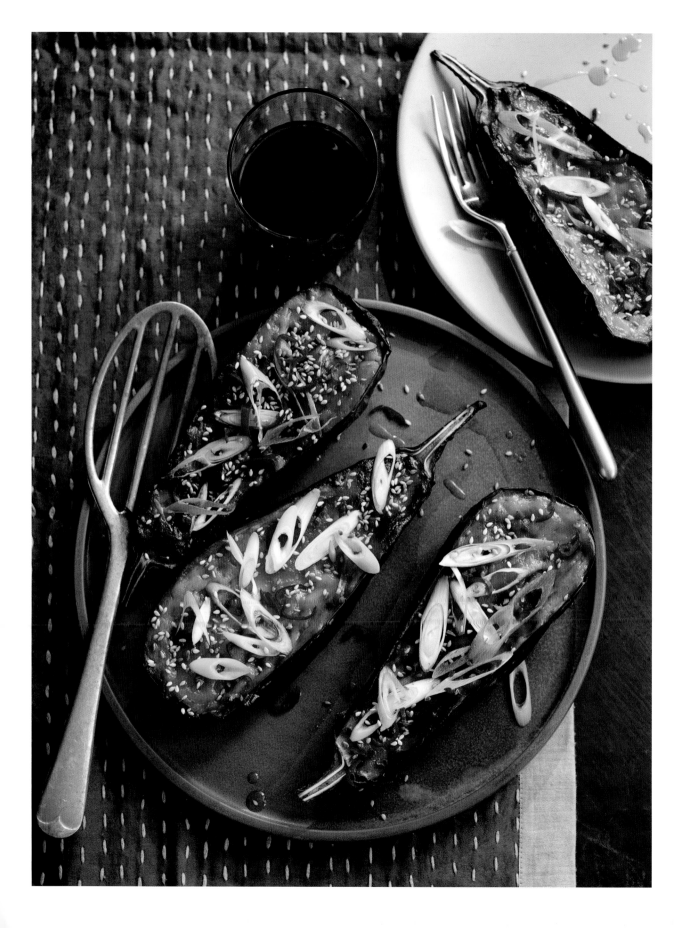

A special thanks to my mate Mai-yee for this recipe, the perfect starter to any oriental meal. The ingredients are readily available in major supermarkets or oriental food stores. You will need white miso paste as there's no substitute, but you can use dry sherry for sake, very sweet sherry or 1 tablespoon rice wine with 1 teaspoon caster/superfine sugar for mirin, and vegetable or chicken stock for dashi, if necessary.

Baked Miso Aubergine

MAKES 4 adult portions
PREPARATION TIME 5 minutes
COOKING TIME 35 minutes

1 tbsp sake
1 tbsp mirin
100g/3½oz white miso paste
1 egg yolk
1 tbsp caster/superfine sugar
4 tbsp dashi stock
2 aubergines/eggplants
sunflower oil, for brushing
sesame oil, for drizzling

TO SERVE
2 tsp toasted sesame seeds
4 spring onions/scallions, finely sliced
½ red chilli, deseeded and finely sliced

1 Preheat the oven to 200°C/400°F/gas 6 and line a baking sheet with baking paper.

2 Put the sake and mirin in a small saucepan over a medium heat and bring just to the boil. Cook for about 30 seconds for the alcohol to burn off. Reduce the heat to low and, using a small whisk, mix in the miso, egg yolk and sugar. Add the stock and cook gently for about 5 minutes until you have the consistency of custard, stirring frequently. Remove from the heat. (This thick miso sauce can be made a day ahead and kept covered in the refrigerator.)

3 Cut the aubergines/eggplants in half lengthways and, using a small, sharp knife, diagonally score lines into the flesh, about 1cm/½in apart, to form a lattice pattern, taking care not to cut all the way through. Brush both sides of the aubergine/eggplant with the sunflower oil and put, cut-side down, on the prepared baking sheet. Bake for 15 minutes, then turn the aubergines/eggplants over, return to the oven and cook for a further 10 minutes or so until the aubergine/eggplant flesh is soft and golden.

4 Preheat the grill/broiler to high. Remove the aubergines/eggplants from the oven and drizzle with sesame oil. Spread the miso sauce on top, then grill/broil for a couple of minutes until the sauce bubbles.

5 Serve hot, scattered with the sesame seeds, spring onions/scallions and red chilli, and enjoy straight away.

Lifesavers for oriental recipes
sake, mirin and miso marinade
Once you have these ingredients you'll find many uses for them in stir-fries and marinades for a variety of oriental recipes. A tasty marinade I like to make is to mix together **4 tbsp sake**, **4 tbsp mirin**, **120g/4¼oz white miso paste** and **60g/2¼oz/heaped ¼ cup caster/superfine sugar**. It can be used to marinate fish or chicken (for at least 24 hours) before grilling/broiling or oven baking. Both kids and adults will love the sweet flavour it creates.

A deliciously simple dish made with coconut milk for a rich finish. You can make the whole thing a day or two in advance, or split up the stages, and marinate the chicken and make the tomato sauce the day before, then cook the finished dish on the day you need it.

South Indian Chicken Curry

MAKES 4 adult portions
PREPARATION TIME 15 minutes, plus at least 10 minutes marinating
COOKING TIME 1 hour

8–12 skinless, boneless chicken thighs (depending on size)
1 tsp turmeric
1 tsp ground coriander
1 tsp hot chilli powder
½ tsp coarsely and freshly ground black pepper
juice of 1 lemon
4 tbsp sunflower oil
1 tsp black mustard seeds
2 large pinches of dried curry leaves
1 large onion, sliced
2cm/¾in piece of root ginger, peeled and grated
3 garlic cloves, crushed
400g/14oz/1¾ cups canned chopped tomatoes
400ml/14fl oz/scant 1¾ cups canned coconut milk
1½ tbsp tamarind paste
1 handful of coriander/cilantro leaves, roughly chopped
sea salt

TO SERVE
Perfect Basmati Rice (see page 14)
naan bread (optional)

1 Put the chicken in a large freezer bag. Mix together the turmeric, ground coriander, chilli powder, black pepper and lemon juice, then pour over the chicken. Seal the bag and mix everything together. Leave to marinate in the refrigerator for at least 10 minutes but, for a better flavour, an hour or longer is preferable.

2 Heat 2 tbsp of the oil in a saucepan over a medium heat and add the mustard seeds and curry leaves. When the mustard seeds begin to pop about, stir in the onion. Cover and cook for 10–15 minutes, stirring occasionally. Add the ginger and garlic and cook for a couple of minutes. Stir in the tomatoes and 200ml/7fl oz/scant 1 cup water. The best thing to do is half fill the empty tomato can with water and pour straight into the pan. Bring to the boil, then reduce the heat and leave to simmer for about 15 minutes.

3 Meanwhile, heat the remaining oil in a large saucepan or flameproof casserole over a medium heat. When almost smoking, add the marinated chicken, with any marinade, and cook for about 8 minutes until the chicken is golden all over. Stir in the tomato sauce, coconut milk, tamarind and a good pinch of salt. Bring to the boil, then reduce the heat and leave to simmer for 25–30 minutes until the chicken is tender and cooked through and the sauce thick. Stir in the chopped coriander/cilantro and serve with rice and naan bread, if you like.

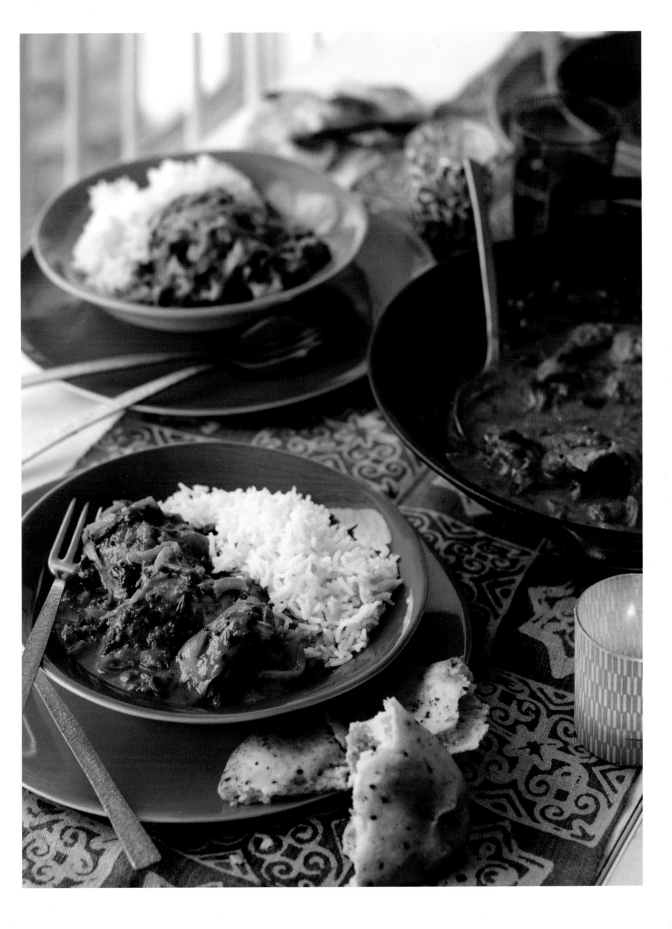

This is a lovely, simple summery recipe that can easily be transformed into a vegetarian dish by swapping the duck for sliced, pan-fried halloumi cheese. The lentil salad is delicious the following day, and if you mix it with crumbled feta, it makes a perfect packed lunch or quick, healthy snack.

Honey and Cinnamon Duck with Lentil and Pomegranate Salad

MAKES 4 adult portions
PREPARATION TIME 15 minutes
COOKING TIME 18 minutes

FOR THE HONEY AND CINNAMON DUCK
4 duck breasts, skin on
2 tsp cinnamon
2 tbsp olive oil
3 tbsp clear honey
sea salt and freshly ground black pepper

FOR THE LENTIL AND POMEGRANATE SALAD
500g/1lb 2oz cooked Puy lentils (see below)
1 red onion, finely sliced
100g/3½oz baby spinach leaves
1 small bunch mint, roughly chopped
1 pomegranate (or use a 100g/3½oz tub ready-prepared seeds)
juice of 1 lemon
3 tbsp extra virgin olive oil
½ tsp ground cumin
¼ tsp ground coriander
75g/2½oz/scant ½ cup toasted almonds

FOR THE SPICED YOGURT
1–2 tsp harissa paste
6 tbsp Greek yogurt

1 Preheat the oven to 190°C/375°F/gas 5.

2 Score the duck skin with a sharp knife several times, then rub the cinnamon and some salt and pepper into the skin and meat. Heat the oil in an ovenproof frying pan over a medium heat, add the duck, skin-side down, and cook for 10 minutes until crispy. Drain off the fat, turn the duck breasts over and drizzle the honey over the skin. Transfer to the oven for 8 minutes, then remove from the pan and leave to rest in a warm place for at least 5 minutes.

3 In a large bowl, mix together the lentils, onion, spinach leaves and mint. Cut the pomegranates in half and, holding each half over the bowl, bash the outer skin with a wooden spoon until all the seeds fall into the bowl. You'll need to bash the skin a few times before the seeds begin to fall out, but they will. Mix the ingredients together.

4 In a separate bowl, mix together the lemon juice, extra virgin olive oil, cumin and coriander/cilantro, and season with salt and pepper. Pour over the salad and mix well. Sprinkle with the almonds. Mix together the harissa paste and yogurt.

5 Serve the duck whole or sliced, with the lentil salad and spiced yogurt.

How to cook

puy lentils
Shop-bought packs of ready-to-eat Puy lentils are an ideal time-saver for this recipe but if you are cooking your own, here's how to do it. To make 500g/1lb 2oz cooked lentils, rinse **250g/9oz/1¼ cups dried Puy lentils** under running water. Put in a saucepan and cover with 3 times their volume (about **750ml/26fl oz/3 cups**) **hot vegetable stock**. Bring to the boil, then reduce the heat and leave to simmer for 20–25 minutes, or perhaps a little longer, until just tender. Drain and serve or leave to cool.

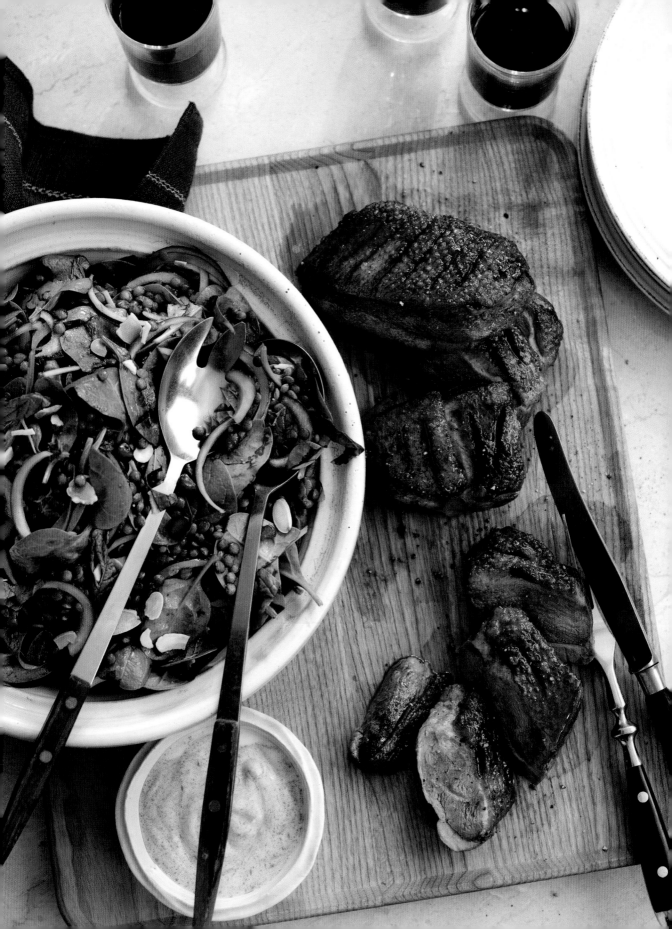

Crispy Pork Belly with Warm Bean, Fennel and Apple Salad

MAKES 4 adult portions
PREPARATION TIME 25 minutes,
   plus 30 minutes resting
COOKING TIME 3 hours

FOR THE PORK
1.5–1.75kg/3lb 5oz–3lb 13oz piece
   of boneless pork belly, scored
2 tsp flaked sea salt
olive oil, for drizzling
2 tsp fennel seeds, crushed
juice of 1 lemon

FOR THE WARM BEAN, FENNEL AND
   APPLE SALAD
2 tbsp olive oil
2 fennel bulbs, finely sliced
250g/9oz green beans, cut into short
   sticks
2 red-skinned apples, cored and cut into
   about 1cm/½in chunks
a pinch of dried chilli/hot pepper flakes
750g/1lb 10oz canned cannellini beans,
   drained
200ml/7fl oz/scant 1 cup chicken stock
a squeeze of lemon juice
sea salt and freshly ground black pepper

1 For really crisp crackling, rub the pork skin generously with the salt, put the pork skin-side down on a wire rack in a roasting pan, cover and leave in the refrigerator overnight to draw out excess moisture.

2 Preheat the oven to 240°C/475°F/gas 8. Pat the pork dry with paper towels. Put skin-side up in a roasting pan. Drizzle a little olive oil over the skin, then rub in the fennel seeds and sea salt, making sure they go down between the score lines. Roast for 30 minutes.

3 Pour the lemon juice over the meat. Reduce the oven temperature to 160°C/315°F/gas 2–3 and cook for a further 1½–2 hours, checking twice during that time that the pork fat and juices are not burning on the base of the pan. If they are, just add a cup of water. At the end of the cooking time, the meat will be meltingly soft and the skin wonderfully crisp. Continue to roast the pork if you want the skin even crispier; it won't do the meat any harm. Transfer the pork to a board, cover loosely with foil and leave to rest in a warm place for up to 30 minutes.

4 When you are almost ready to serve, throw together the warm salad. Heat the oil in a large frying pan over a medium heat, add the fennel and green beans and fry for about 8 minutes until just tender. Add the apples and chilli/hot pepper flakes and cook for about 2 minutes until just tender. Stir in the cannellini beans and stock. Bring to the boil, then reduce the heat and leave to simmer for 2 minutes until the beans are heated through. Season lightly with salt, pepper and a squeeze of lemon juice.

5 Cut the pork into large pieces, using a serrated knife, and serve with the warm bean salad.

Leftovers for tortillas
pork and hoisin wrap
Shred any **leftover pork** into pieces. Spread **a tortilla wrap** with **1 tbsp hoisin sauce**, then top with the pork, some **shredded crispy lettuce**, **chopped spring onion/scallion** and **matchsticks of cucumber**. Roll and enjoy straight away, or, if you're making it for a packed lunch, wrap in a sheet of baking paper with the ends twisted to resemble a cracker.

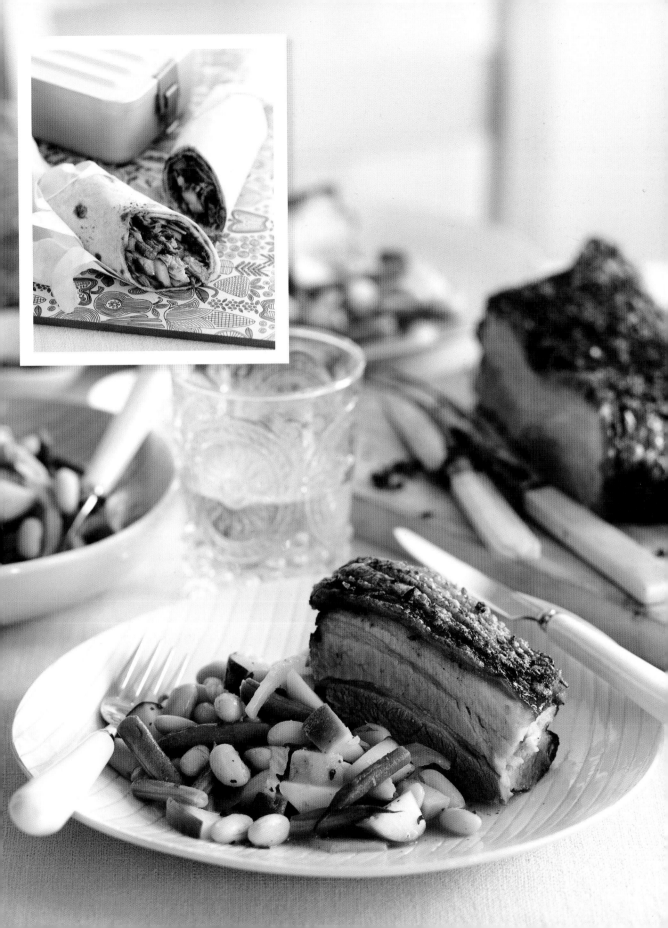

This is a delicious North African dish that is ideally suited to serving with couscous or flatbread. You need two lovely juicy lemons – buy the unwaxed ones if you can. It's a great dish to choose for a dinner party because you can make it the day before.

Moroccan Lamb Meatballs with Olives and Lemon

MAKES 4 adult portions
PREPARATION TIME 20 minutes
COOKING TIME 40 minutes

3 onions, quartered
500g/1lb 2oz minced/ground lamb
1 tsp ground cinnamon
1 tsp ground cumin
½ tsp cayenne pepper
finely grated zest and juice of 1 lemon, plus 1 lemon, cut into wedges
1 handful of flat-leaf parsley leaves, chopped
2 tbsp olive oil
1 red chilli, deseeded and finely chopped
25g/1oz root ginger, peeled and grated or finely chopped
a large pinch of saffron strands
250ml/9fl oz/1 cup lamb stock
2 tbsp tomato purée/paste
100g/3½oz/¾ cup black or green kalamata olives, pitted
1 small handful of coriander/cilantro leaves, chopped
sea salt and freshly ground black pepper
couscous or flatbread, to serve

1 Put the onions in a food processor and whizz until finely chopped. Remove half and leave to one side. Add the lamb, spices, lemon zest, parsley and salt and pepper to the food processor and whizz to combine. Tip out the mixture and, using wet hands to stop the mixture sticking to you, shape it into walnut-sized balls. (The meatballs can be made a day ahead of cooking and kept in the refrigerator. Or, to be mega ahead of time, they can be frozen for up to 3 months.)

2 Heat the oil in a large flameproof casserole over a medium heat, add the reserved onion, the chilli, ginger and saffron and cook for about 5 minutes until the onion is softened and starting to colour. Add the lemon juice, stock, tomato purée/paste and olives and bring to the boil. Add the meatballs, reduce the heat and cover with a lid. Cook for 20 minutes. (You can make the recipe to this point the day before, then finish it from here when you like.)

3 Remove the lid and add the coriander/cilantro and lemon wedges, tucking them into the dish. Cook without the lid for a further 10 minutes until the liquid has reduced and thickened slightly.

4 Serve hot with couscous or flatbread.

Bulghar wheat or brown rice go really well with this delicious dish of meltingly tender lamb with that wonderful sweet-spicy combination of Middle Eastern cuisine. But the best thing about this dish is that you can cook it completely the day before, making it the ideal dinner party dish when you know you'll have very little time to cook on the actual day.

Persian Lamb Stew

MAKES 4 adult portions
PREPARATION TIME 15 minutes
COOKING TIME 2¼ hours

100g/3½oz/⅔ cup walnut halves or
   pieces
2 tbsp olive oil
2 onions, sliced
2 garlic cloves, crushed
800g–1kg/1lb 12oz–2lb 4oz lamb
   shoulder, diced
½ tsp turmeric
½ tsp ground cinnamon
100g/3½oz/scant 1 cup dried
   cranberries
500ml/17fl oz/2 cups lamb stock
4 tbsp pomegranate molasses
1 small bunch flat-leaf parsley, chopped
sea salt and freshly ground black pepper

1 Preheat the oven to 150°C/300°F/gas 2.

2 Put the walnuts on a baking sheet and bake for about 10 minutes until toasted. Leave to cool slightly, then tip into a sandwich bag and bash with a rolling pin to crush finely, or chop them on a board.

3 Heat the oil in a large, flameproof casserole over a medium heat, add the onions and cook for 10 minutes until softened and golden. Increase the heat to high, add the garlic and lamb and cook until browned all over. Stir in the spices and cook for about 1 minute. Mix in the cranberries, stock, pomegranate molasses and walnuts. Cover with a lid and bake for 1½ hours.

4 Remove the lid and cook for a further 15–30 minutes until the sauce has thickened slightly. (The stew can be cooked to this point at least a day beforehand and gently reheated when needed.)

5 Season to taste with salt and pepper, stir in the parsley and serve.

Leftovers for dessert
pomegranate and yogurt puddings

This is a lovely, refreshing dessert to serve after the Persian Lamb Stew. To serve 4, layer up **segments of 3 oranges, 25g/1oz roughly chopped pistachio nuts, 250ml/9floz/1 cup Greek yogurt** and **drizzles of pomegranate molasses** (roughly **1 tbsp** per serving) in glasses or small dishes. Finish with **a scattering of pistachios** and **mint sprigs** to decorate.

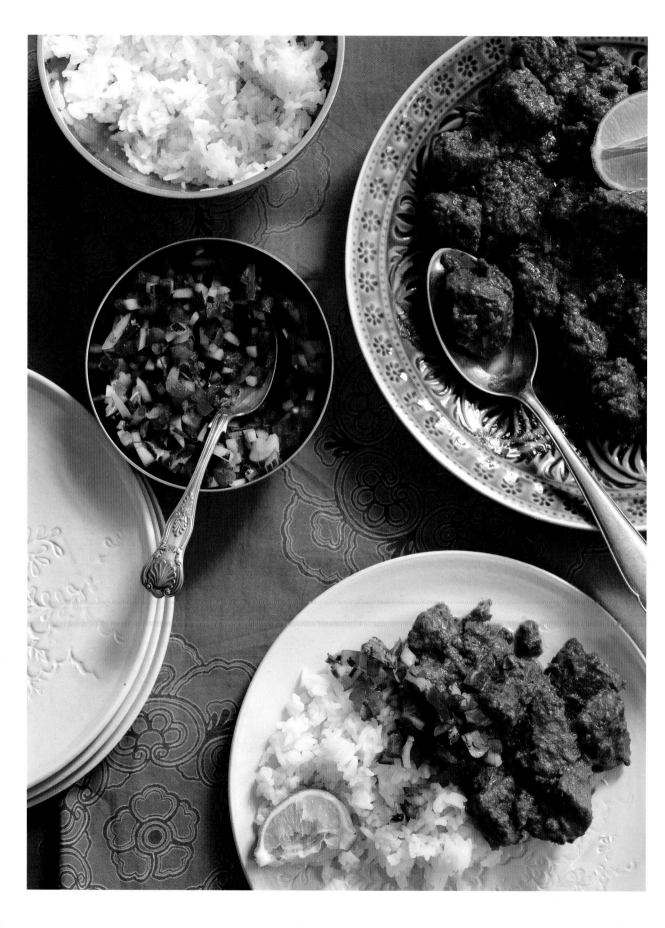

This delicious Indonesian coconut beef curry needs to simmer for about three hours, which gives you plenty of time to get on with doing the one hundred things you have to do before people start arriving.

Beef Rendang

MAKES 4 adult portions
PREPARATION TIME 20 minutes
COOKING TIME 3½ hours

4 shallots, roughly chopped
3 garlic cloves
3cm/1¼in piece of root ginger, peeled
  and roughly chopped
3 red chillies, 2 deseeded and all
  3 roughly chopped
2cm/¾in piece of galangal (if available,
  if not, add a little more ginger)
1 lemongrass stalk, roughly chopped
1 tsp ground turmeric
1½ tsp sea salt
1kg/2lb 4oz stewing or casserole beef
800ml/28fl oz/scant 3½ cups canned
  coconut milk
3 kaffir lime leaves (fresh or dried),
  chopped or crushed

**FOR THE TOMATO AND CORIANDER
  SALSA**
3 ripe tomatoes, quartered, deseeded
  and finely diced
¼ cucumber, finely diced
1 small red onion, finely diced
1 handful of coriander/cilantro leaves,
  chopped
juice of ½ lime
1½ tbsp olive oil
sea salt and freshly ground black pepper

TO SERVE
lime wedges
boiled or steamed Thai Jasmine rice

1 Put the shallots, garlic, ginger, chillies, galangal, if using, lemongrass, turmeric and salt in a blender or food processor and add 150ml/5fl oz/ scant ⅔ cup water. Blitz to a smooth paste.

2 Put the spice paste in a large wok or saucepan, add the beef, coconut milk and lime leaves. Top up with water if the meat is not quite covered. Stir well and bring to the boil over a medium heat, then reduce to a simmer and leave to gently bubble away for 3–3½ hours, stirring occasionally.

3 Make the salsa by mixing together the tomatoes, cucumber, onion and coriander/cilantro. Keep in the refrigerator until you are ready to serve. (You can make this a few hours ahead of time, if you like.)

4 When the dish is ready, the coconut milk will have reduced, with the oil starting to appear on the surface, and the curry will be fairly thick. (This dish can be cooked the day before and gently reheated when needed.)

5 Drizzle the lime juice and olive oil over the salsa, season with salt and pepper and toss together.

6 Serve the beef hot with lime wedges, Thai rice and the tomato salsa.

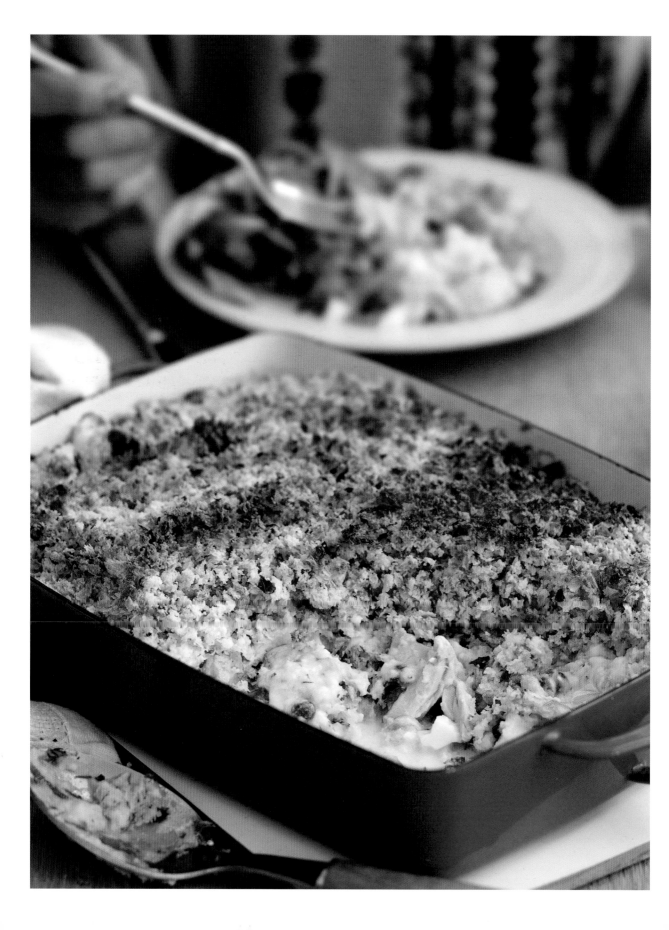

Everyone loves a fish pie so I make extra for the kids, but to ring the changes from a traditional potato-topped pie, I make this with a crunchy, cheesy topping. It always goes down a treat. As an added bonus, it's quicker and easier to make than a traditional mashed potato topping.

Salmon and Seafood Crumble

MAKES 4 adult and 2 kid-sized portions
PREPARATION TIME 20 minutes
COOKING TIME 55 minutes

FOR THE FILLING
75g/2½oz butter
1 onion, chopped
1 bay leaf
50g/1¾oz/scant ½ cup plain/all-purpose flour
150ml/5fl oz/scant ⅔ cup white wine
200ml/7fl oz/scant 1 cup milk
750g/1lb 10oz salmon fillet, cut into 3cm/1¼in cubes
300g/10½oz raw, peeled tiger prawns/ jumbo shrimp
3 eggs, hard-boiled and chopped
2 tbsp chopped dill
2 tbsp capers
sea salt and freshly ground black pepper

FOR THE CRUMBLE TOPPING
1 ciabatta loaf, about 200g/7oz
25g/1oz/¼ cup finely grated Parmesan cheese
3 tbsp olive oil
2 tbsp chopped parsley leaves

1 Preheat the oven to 200°C/400°F/gas 6.

2 Melt the butter in a large saucepan over a medium heat, add the onion and the bay leaf and fry until the onion is softened but not coloured. Stir in the flour for about 30 seconds, then gradually add the wine, stirring continuously to prevent any floury lumps, then finally stir in the milk. Bring to the boil, then reduce the heat and simmer for a few minutes until you have a thick sauce, still stirring. Stir in the salmon and prawns/ shrimp and cook for a few minutes until the prawns/shrimp turn pink. Add the eggs and dill, and season with salt and pepper.

3 Spoon the majority of the mixture into a large ovenproof dish and scatter over the capers. Divide the remaining filling between two small pots for the kids. You can add extra capers to theirs, too, if you think they will like them.

4 To make the topping, tear the ciabatta into pieces, put in a food processor and blitz to a rough crumb. Add the Parmesan, oil and parsley, then briefly blitz to combine. (The filling and crumbs can be made a day in advance and kept in the refrigerator.)

5 When you are ready to cook the crumble, scatter the topping over the filling, put the dish on a baking sheet and bake for 30–40 minutes (or slightly longer if you are cooking the filling from chilled) until the topping is golden and the filling is bubbling at the edges. Serve the crumble piping hot.

Thai Tuna Fishcakes with Sweet and Sour Dipping Sauce and Rice Salad

MAKES 4 adult portions
PREPARATION TIME 30 minutes
COOKING TIME 6 minutes

FOR THE RICE SALAD
300g/10½oz/1½ cups Thai Jasmine rice
  or basmati rice
4 tbsp rice vinegar
2 tbsp caster/superfine sugar
1 bunch spring onions/scallions, finely
  sliced
1 red pepper, deseeded and finely sliced
½ cucumber, halved lengthways,
  deseeded and finely sliced
1 large handful each of basil, mint and
  coriander/cilantro leaves
sea salt

FOR THE THAI TUNA FISHCAKES
600g/1lb 5oz fresh tuna
1½ tbsp Thai red curry paste
1½ tbsp Thai fish sauce
1 handful of coriander/cilantro leaves
4 spring onions/scallions, roughly
  chopped
1 egg, lightly beaten
sunflower oil, for frying

**FOR THE SWEET AND SOUR DIPPING
  SAUCE**
1 red chilli, deseeded and finely
  chopped
4 tbsp rice vinegar
4 tsp caster/superfine sugar
1cm/½in piece of root ginger, peeled
  and grated
2 tbsp finely chopped coriander/cilantro
  leaves

1 To make the salad, put the rice in a saucepan with a pinch of salt and 400ml/14fl oz/scant 1¾ cups water. Bring to the boil, then cover with a tight-fitting lid, reduce the heat to low and leave the rice to cook for 10 minutes. Remove the pan from the heat but don't lift the lid. Leave the rice to stand for a further 5–10 minutes.

2 Fluff up the rice with a fork, tip out on to a baking sheet, loosely spreading it to cool it down, and leave to cool for 5 minutes to reach room temperature. Put in the refrigerator to chill.

3 Once the rice is cold, transfer it to a large bowl. Gently heat the rice vinegar, sugar and a pinch of salt in a small pan, stirring until the sugar has dissolved. Stir into the rice with the spring onions/scallions, red pepper, cucumber and herbs. The salad is ready.

4 Put all the fishcake ingredients in a food processor and blitz briefly to a smooth paste. Using wet hands to stop the mixture sticking to you, divide into about 12 balls and flatten each one lightly to form a patty.

5 Mix together all the ingredients for the dipping sauce. (You can prepare everything to this point a good few hours in advance and keep it the refrigerator.)

6 Heat about 1cm/½in oil in a frying pan over a medium heat, add the fishcakes and fry in batches for about 3 minutes on each side until golden. Drain on paper towels and serve with the rice salad and a bowl of dipping sauce.

Leftovers transformed
simple sushi
Making sushi is much simpler than you might think. Chill any leftover rice salad well. With wet hands, gently shape a ball of rice the size of a small egg into an oblong. Snip large pieces of **red pepper** or **cucumber** with scissors. Dot a little **wasabi paste** (or mayonnaise) on the surface and finish by topping with a **cooked prawn/shrimp**, **smoked salmon**, **crab stick**, **canned tuna** mashed with some **mayonnaise**, **sliced avocado**, **cooked asparagus tip** or, if you just happen to randomly have any, some fresh **slices of salmon** or **tuna**. Serve with **soy sauce**, **wasabi** and **pickled ginger** for a proper sushi experience.

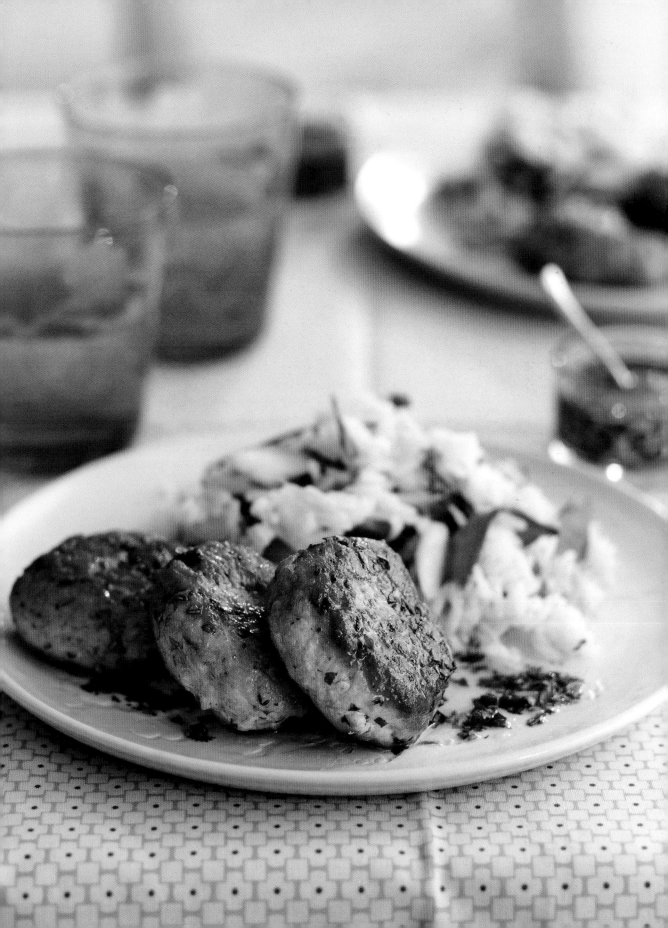

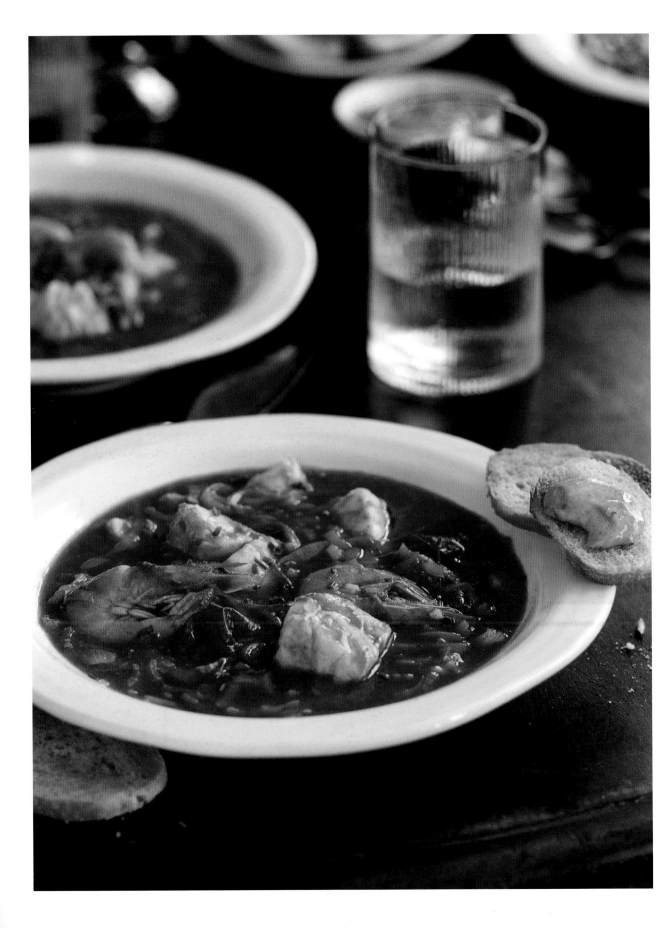

To save a huge amount of time and effort, this recipe has a secret short cut: it uses a can of seafood soup as its base. But if you don't tell anyone, they will never know.

Effortless Bouillabaisse

MAKES 4 adult portions
PREPARATION TIME 20 minutes
COOKING TIME 20 minutes

FOR THE BOUILLABAISSE
2 tbsp olive oil
2 leeks, thinly sliced
400g/14oz canned cherry tomatoes
400g/14oz canned lobster or seafood bisque
2 peeled strips of orange zest
a large pinch of dried chilli/hot pepper flakes
a small splash of brandy
1kg/2lb 4oz white fish, such as monkfish, cod, pollack, haddock or sea bass, cut into large bite-size pieces
8–12 raw, whole king prawns/jumbo shrimp
1 tbsp chopped flat-leaf parsley leaves
1 tbsp chopped chives
sea salt and freshly ground black pepper

FOR THE TOAST
8 slices of French baguette, for toasting
extra virgin olive oil, for drizzling
6 tbsp garlic mayonnaise
1 tsp harissa paste

1 Heat the olive oil in a large saucepan over a medium heat, add the leeks and fry for a few minutes until they are softened but not coloured. Add the tomatoes, bisque, orange zest, chilli/hot pepper flakes, brandy and 150ml/5fl oz/scant ⅔ cup water. Bring to the boil, then reduce the heat and leave to simmer for 5 minutes. Stir the fish into the pan, return to a simmer and cook for 8 minutes. Add the prawns/shrimp, stirring in gently. Return to a simmer and cook for about 3 minutes, or until the prawns/shrimp have turned pink.

2 Meanwhile, to make the toast, drizzle the bread with a little extra virgin olive oil, then lightly toast on both sides. Mix together the garlic mayonnaise and harissa paste. Either spread the spiced mayonnaise on the toast or spoon into a bowl.

3 Once all the fish is cooked, season lightly with salt and pepper and remove the orange zest strips if you can find them. Scatter with the parsley and chives.

4 Spoon the bouillabaisse into bowls and serve with the toast and garlic mayonnaise.

Leftovers for a marinade
harissa and yogurt marinade
If you are stuck for a quick and simple way to liven up chicken breast or fish fillet during the week, grab your open jar of harissa and try this out. Mix together **2 tsp harissa** with **2 tbsp Greek** or **plain yogurt,** the **grated zest and juice of ½ lemon**, **½ tsp ground cumin** and **a pinch of salt**. Spread or rub all over **2 scored chicken breasts** or **2 fish fillets** or **steaks**, cover and leave to marinate in the refrigerator for anything between 10 minutes and 24 hours.

This is my idea of a real-life recipe: a paella dish that doesn't require you to invest in a vast frying pan, or expect you to be fiddling about in the kitchen while your guests catch up on the must-hear gossip.

Baked Seafood Paella

MAKES 4 adult portions
PREPARATION TIME 20 minutes
COOKING TIME 30 minutes

3 tbsp olive oil
1 onion, chopped
2 garlic cloves, crushed
1 red pepper, deseeded and sliced
300g/10½oz/1⅓ cups paella rice
250ml/9fl oz/1 cup dry white wine
a large pinch of saffron strands
1 tsp smoked Spanish paprika or
    standard sweet paprika
750ml/26fl oz/3 cups hot fish or chicken
    stock
500g/1lb 2oz shellfish, such as mussels
    and/or clams
2 medium squid tubes, cut into rings
150g/5½oz/scant 1 cup frozen peas,
    defrosted, or fresh green beans,
    chopped
8–12 raw, whole king prawns/jumbo
    shrimp
½ small bunch flat-leaf parsley, chopped
1 lemon, cut into wedges
sea salt and freshly ground black pepper

1 Scrub the mussels thoroughly with a stiff brush under cold running water to remove all traces of grit, then remove any barnacles or other debris attached to the shells and pull off and discard any beards. Rinse again and discard any mussels that stay open.

2 Preheat the oven to 220°C/425°F/gas 7.

3 Heat the oil in a large flameproof casserole over a medium heat, add the onion, garlic and red pepper and fry for about 5 minutes until the onion has softened. Stir in the rice for a minute or so until it is coated in the oil, then add the wine, saffron, paprika and stock. Stir well and bring to the boil, then bake, uncovered, for 15 minutes.

4 Stir in the mussels and/or clams, squid and peas and season lightly with salt and pepper. Nestle the prawns/shrimp into the surface. Return to the oven and cook for a further 10 minutes until the rice is tender and the seafood is cooked through. Make sure all the prawns/shrimp are pink and discard any mussel or clam shells that haven't opened.

5 Sprinkle over the parsley and serve with lemon wedges. Provide empty bowls for the shells, and a few finger bowls of warm water and plenty of napkins for messy fingers.

How to make

paella mixta

If your friends aren't massively into seafood, then make your paella with chicken and chorizo. Add **150g/5½oz thickly sliced or chopped chorizo** and **4 roughly chopped chicken thighs** to the **fried onion** and cook until the chicken is golden. Add the **rice** and follow the recipe as above, but just using **prawns/shrimp** and not the mussels or squid.

A bowl of fluffy basmati rice and some Cucumber Raita (see page 25) make the perfect dishes to serve with this medium-hot curry. For a milder flavour, remove the chilli seeds before chopping.

Healthy Vegetable Dhansak

MAKES 4 adult portions
PREPARATION TIME 25 minutes
COOKING TIME 45 minutes

200g/7oz/scant 1 cup red lentils
1 large onion
4 garlic cloves
3 green chillies, stalks removed
2.5cm/1in piece of root ginger, peeled
3 tbsp sunflower oil
2 sweet potatoes, peeled and diced into bite-size cubes
2 large carrots, peeled and diced
2 red peppers, deseeded and diced
150g/5½oz/scant 1¼ cups sultanas/ golden raisins
½ tsp turmeric
1 tsp ground cumin
1 tsp ground coriander
1l/35fl oz/4 cups hot vegetable stock
2 tbsp tomato purée/paste
4 large ripe tomatoes, each cut into 8 wedges
200g/7oz green beans, halved
2 tsp garam masala
1 small bunch coriander/cilantro, chopped
sea salt
pickles or condiments of your choice, to serve

1 Put the lentils in a bowl of cold water and leave to soak for about 3 minutes. Drain and leave to one side.

2 Put the onion, garlic, chillies and ginger in a food processor and pulse until finely chopped.

3 Heat the oil in a large saucepan over a medium heat, add the onion mixture and fry for about 5 minutes until it is starting to soften and become golden. Add the sweet potatoes, carrots and red peppers and fry for about 5 minutes. Stir in the sultanas/golden raisins, turmeric, cumin and ground coriander and cook for about 1 minute. Add the drained lentils, hot stock, tomato purée/paste and tomatoes. Stir well and cover with a lid. Simmer for 20 minutes, stirring a couple of times. (The dhansak can be cooked up to this stage and removed from the heat at least 2 hours before needed. Simply return to the simmer and continue cooking for 10–15 minutes before serving.)

4 Add the green beans and garam masala, then simmer with the lid off for a further 10–15 minutes until all the vegetables are cooked through and tender. Sprinkle with the coriander/cilantro.

5 Season with a pinch of salt and serve as it is or with pickles or condiments of your choice.

Leftovers for a liquid lunch
dhansak soup
Any leftover dhansak is great made into a soup. All you need to do is blend or liquidize with enough **vegetable stock** to loosen to a soup consistency, then heat gently until simmering. Re-season with **salt** if needed and serve. To spoon on top of the soup, I like to fry some **sliced onions** and a **few black mustard seeds** in **sunflower oil** until the onions are soft, golden and sweet.

Quinoa, Beetroot, Squash and Feta Salad

MAKES 4 adult portions
PREPARATION TIME 25 minutes, plus
   cooling
COOKING TIME 50 minutes

**FOR THE QUINOA, BEETROOT, SQUASH
   AND FETA SALAD**
1 butternut squash, peeled, deseeded
   and cut into bite-size wedges
4 raw beetroot, cut into bite-size wedges
2 tbsp olive oil
60g/2¼oz/scant ½ cup hazelnuts
100g/3½oz/½ cup quinoa
150g/5½oz baby spinach leaves
1 small bunch mint leaves, roughly
   chopped
1 bunch spring onions/scallions, finely
   sliced
1 red chilli, deseeded and finely sliced
400g/14oz feta cheese, crumbled
sea salt and freshly ground black pepper

**FOR THE HONEY AND MUSTARD
   DRESSING**
4 tbsp rapeseed/canola oil
2 tbsp clear honey
2 tbsp white wine vinegar
1 tbsp Dijon mustard
finely grated zest of 1 orange

1 Preheat the oven to 200°C/400°F/gas 6.

2 Put the butternut squash and beetroot in a roasting pan, toss in the oil and season lightly with salt and pepper. Roast for about 40–50 minutes until they are softened and becoming golden. Once cooked, leave to cool to room temperature.

3 While you are roasting the vegetables, put the hazelnuts in a small baking sheet and roast for 8 minutes until golden. Leave to cool slightly, then roughly chop and leave to one side.

4 Rinse the quinoa in cold water, then put in a saucepan with 300ml/ 10½fl oz/scant 1¼ cups cold water and a pinch of salt. Bring to the boil, then reduce the heat and leave to simmer for 20 minutes until all the water has been absorbed and the quinoa is light and fluffy. Leave to cool.

5 Put the dressing ingredients in a screw-topped jar, shake well, then leave to one side. (You can roast the vegetables and nuts, make the dressing and cook the quinoa a few hours in advance. Cover and keep in the refrigerator until you are ready to finish.)

6 To finish, put everything except the hazelnuts and feta in a bowl, pour over the dressing and toss together well. Serve sprinkled with the feta and hazelnuts.

Leftovers for a 5-a-day lunch
quinoa with ratatouille
It is a good idea to cook extra quinoa and serve it with some ratatouille or roasted vegetables. If the kids like couscous, they should enjoy it; it has a slightly nuttier flavour, and is really good for you. You can stir the extra into casseroles or sauces once they are cooked to bulk them out and for added nutritional value. To make quinoa ratatouille, lightly fry **1 chopped onion** and **2 crushed garlic cloves** in **2 tbsp olive oil**. Add **1 diced red pepper** and **1 diced yellow or orange pepper**, **2 diced courgettes/zucchini** and **½ diced aubergine/ eggplant**. Cook for 2 minutes, then add **400g/14oz/1¾ cups canned chopped tomatoes**, **2 tbsp tomato ketchup**, **½ tsp mixed dried herbs** and season with a little **sea salt** and **freshly ground black pepper**. Cover with a lid and simmer for 30 minutes. Makes 2 adult and 2 kid-sized portions.

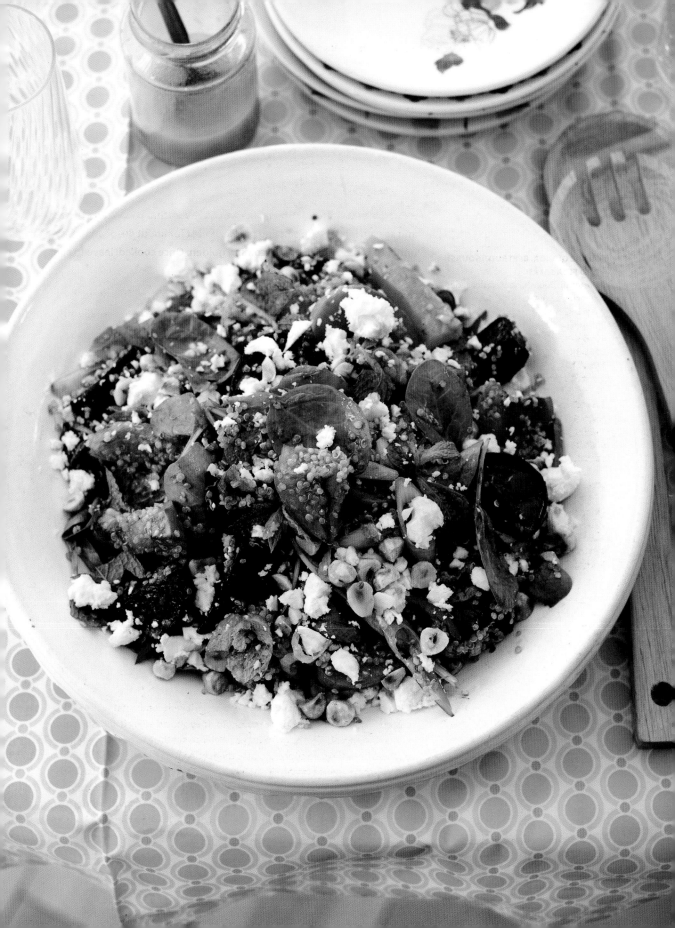

We are in adult territory now so don't let the kids get their hands on any leftovers! If you like, swap the sloe gin for Pimm's and use lemon, orange or strawberry jelly. Try substituting orange segments, strawberries or sliced peaches for the summer berries.

Sloe Gin Jellies with Minted Crème Fraîche

MAKES 4 adult portions
PREPARATION TIME 5 minutes, plus cooling and at least 4 hours setting

FOR THE SLOE GIN JELLIES
375ml/13fl oz/1½ cups apple juice
135g/4¾oz packet of blackcurrant jelly, cut into pieces
200ml/7fl oz/scant 1 cup sloe gin
250g/9oz/1⅔ cups mixed summer berries (blueberries, raspberries, strawberries and blackberries)

FOR THE MINTED CRÈME FRAÎCHE
1 handful of mint leaves, finely chopped, plus extra leaves to decorate
200ml/7fl oz/scant 1 cup half-fat crème fraîche or sour cream
½ lemon
2 tbsp icing/confectioners' sugar, sifted

1 Put 125ml/4fl oz/½ cup of the apple juice in a jug or bowl with the jelly pieces and microwave on high for 1 minute. Remove and stir until the jelly has dissolved. Stir in the remaining apple juice and the sloe gin. Leave to cool.

2 Divide the berries into 4–6 glasses or small dishes and then pour the cooled jelly over the top. Put in the refrigerator to set for at least 4 hours.

3 To make the minted crème fraîche, stir the mint into the crème fraîche with a squeeze of lemon juice and the icing/confectioners' sugar. (The jellies and crème fraîche can be prepared a day in advance and kept in the refrigerator.)

4 Remove the jellies from the refrigerator, decorate with mint leaves and serve with the crème fraîche spooned on top or offered separately.

My other name for this is the Easiest Pud You Could Wish for. Serve it on its own or with some little cookies or shortbread. It's also nice with a mixed berry salad: chopped strawberries, blueberries, raspberries and blackberries tossed in a little icing/confectioners' sugar. You can simply leave out the rosemary or, for a bit of variety, use half lemon and half lime juice. A finely diced ball of stem ginger and 2 tablespoons ginger syrup will spice it up beautifully, while the seeds of 6 cardamom pods infused with the milk, then strained, will give it a new set of flavours.

Lemon and Rosemary Posset

MAKES 4 individual possets
PREPARATION TIME 10 minutes, plus
   cooling and at least 2 hours chilling
COOKING TIME 4 minutes

2 rosemary sprigs
500ml/7fl oz/2 cups double/heavy cream
150g/5½oz/scant ¾ cup caster/superfine
   sugar
80ml/2½fl oz/⅓ cup lemon juice

1 Bruise the rosemary by hitting lightly with a rolling pin (the kids will think you are mad if they see you doing this!) and put in a saucepan with the cream and sugar. Gently bring to the boil. Reduce the heat to low and simmer gently for 3 minutes, stirring occasionally, and making sure it doesn't boil over.

2 Remove from the heat, fish out the rosemary and leave the cream to cool for a few minutes before stirring in the lemon juice.

3 Pour into wine glasses, dishes or cups and leave to cool, then put in the refrigerator for at least 2 hours to chill. (The lemon posset can be made a couple of days before serving and kept covered in the refrigerator.)

Everyone loves a chocolate pudding to round off a delicious meal, so imagine the 'oooohs' you'll get serving three mini ones each. These recipes are simple to put together (two can be made in advance), look great all together on one plate and taste fantastic.

Triple Chocolate Pudding

EACH ONE MAKES 4 adult portions
PREPARATION TIME 10 minutes each, plus chilling

SUPER EASY CHOCOLATE MOUSSE

100g/3½oz dark chocolate, 70% cocoa solids, broken into pieces
100ml/3½fl oz/scant ½ cup double/heavy cream
125ml/4fl oz/½ cup shop-bought or Foolproof Home-made Custard (see page 128)
4 tbsp your favourite liqueur (optional)

1 Put the chocolate in a large, heatproof bowl. Rest the bowl over a pan of gently simmering water, so that the bottom of the bowl does not touch the water. Stir occasionally until the chocolate has melted.

2 Whisk the cream until it just forms soft peaks, then fold in the custard, liqueur, if using, and melted chocolate. Spoon into four espresso cups or little glasses and chill for at least 30 minutes.

BLACK FOREST CREAM CRUNCH

2 tbsp cherry jam
100ml/3½fl oz/scant ½ cup double/heavy cream, lightly whipped
1 tbsp kirsch liqueur or cherry brandy (optional)
100g/3½oz/⅔ cup fresh cherries, pitted, or canned or marinated cherries
4 chocolate cookies, chocolate-coated digestives/Graham crackers or other crunchy cookies, crushed to a crumb
1 tbsp grated dark chocolate, 70% cocoa solids

1 Mix together the cherry jam, whipped cream and kirsch, if using.

2 Layer the mixture with the cherries and cookie crumbs in four small glasses. Chill until needed.

3 When ready to serve, sprinkle with grated chocolate.

BOOZY ICED BERRIES AND HOT WHITE CHOCOLATE SAUCE

250g/9oz mixed frozen berries, defrosted
80ml/2½fl oz/⅓ cup double/heavy cream
80g/2¾oz white chocolate, broken into small pieces
4 tbsp crème de cassis

1 Divide the berries into four small glasses or little plates. Leave in the refrigerator for about 20 minutes before serving.

2 Just before serving, gently melt the cream and chocolate together in a small saucepan or in the microwave.

3 Pour the cassis over the berries, then pour over the white chocolate sauce just as you serve them.

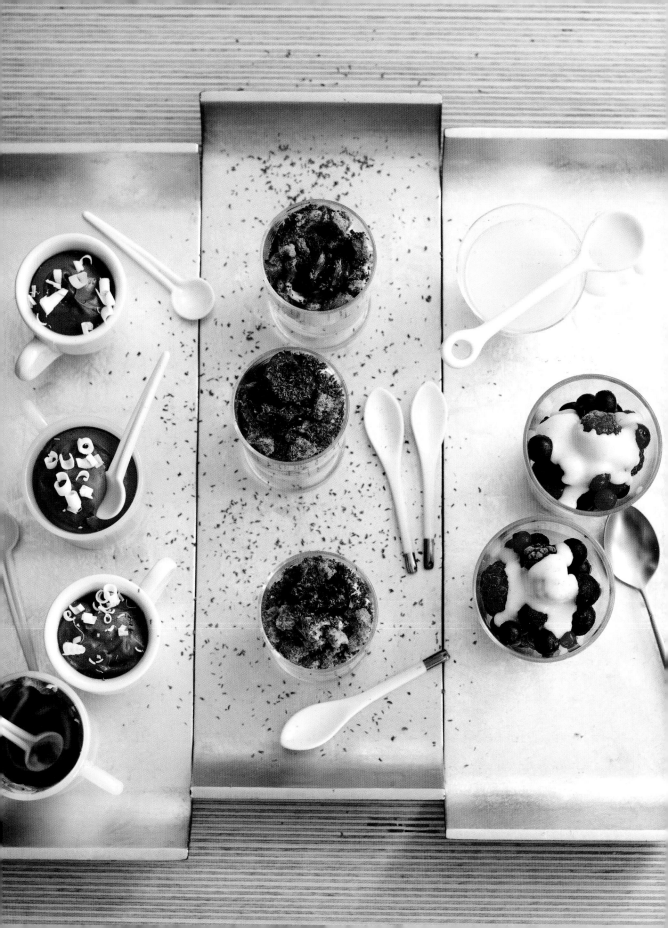

The subtle coconut and orange flavour of these rich creamy panna cottas is perfectly balanced by the tangy, juicy rhubarb, and rounds any meal off perfectly. I like to leave the panna cottas to set in glasses, which saves the hassle of turning them out of moulds when serving, but you can leave to set in lightly greased 200ml/7fl oz teacups, jelly moulds, ramekins or dariole moulds if you prefer.

Coconut and Orange Panna Cotta with Rhubarb

MAKES 4 adult portions
PREPARATION TIME 20 minutes, plus at least 3 hours setting (overnight if possible)
COOKING TIME 35 minutes

FOR THE PANNA COTTA
a little vegetable oil, for greasing
2 tsp powdered gelatine or 4 leaves gelatine
375ml/13fl oz/1½ cups canned coconut milk
200ml/7fl oz/scant 1 cup double/heavy cream
peeled zest of 1 orange
100g/3½oz/scant 1 cup icing/ confectioners' sugar
150ml/5fl oz/scant ⅔ cup plain yogurt

FOR THE RHUBARB
200g/7oz rhubarb, cut into 2cm/1in pieces
55g/2oz/¼ cup caster/superfine sugar
2 tbsp orange juice

1 Put the powdered gelatine in a small dish, sprinkle over 3 tbsp water and leave to absorb the water for 5 minutes. Alternatively, if you are using gelatine leaves, soak them in cold water for 5 minutes to allow them to soften.

2 Put the coconut milk, cream and orange zest in a saucepan over a medium heat and stir in the icing/confectioners' sugar. Gently bring to the boil, stirring occasionally. If you are using leaf gelatine, squeeze out the excess water. Remove the pan from the heat and stir in the gelatine until it has dissolved. Leave to cool for 5 minutes.

3 Stir in the yogurt until smooth, using a whisk if necessary. Strain through a sieve/fine-mesh strainer into a large jug, then pour into the glasses and leave in the refrigerator for 3 hours, or overnight if you can.

4 Preheat the oven to 140°C/275°F/gas 1.

5 To prepare the rhubarb compote, mix together the rhubarb, caster/ superfine sugar and orange juice and put in a roasting pan, laying the rhubarb in a flat layer. Bake for 30 minutes until the rhubarb is tender and the juice is syrupy. Leave to cool. (The panna cottas and the rhubarb can be made a day in advance and kept in the refrigerator.)

6 Spoon some rhubarb on top of the panna cottas with a little of the syrup to serve.

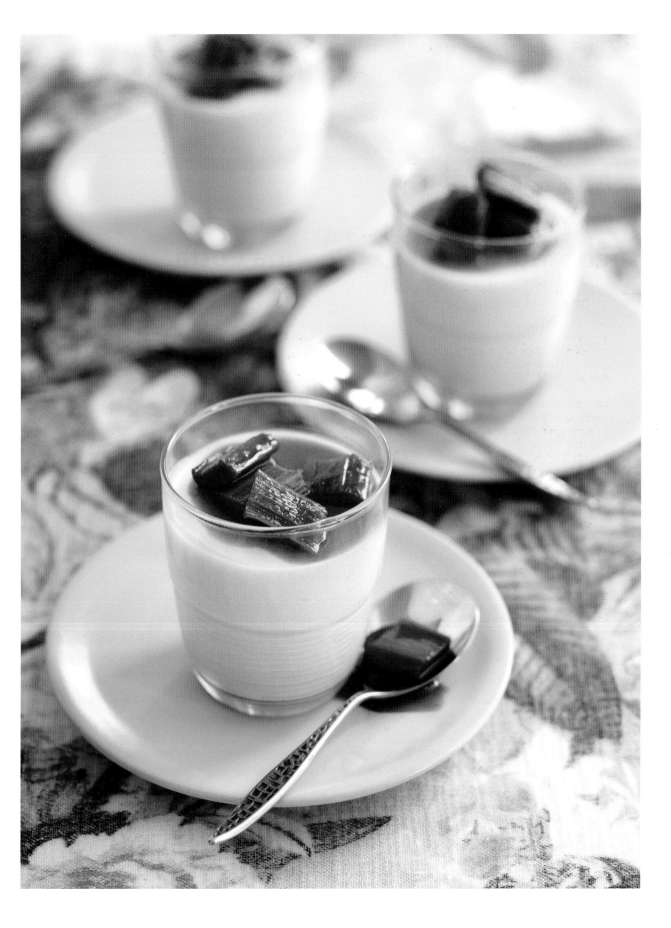

Chocolate and caramel are a match made in heaven but add a little salt to the mix and it takes the flavours to another level. You simply must try this recipe – there are no excuses, as it can easily be made the day before you need it. (If you really are struggling for time, check out the How to below.) This makes a large tart so there's plenty for four adults plus leftovers for the kids.

Chocolate and Salted Caramel Tart

MAKES 23cm/9in tart
PREPARATION TIME 20 minutes, plus
 cooling
COOKING TIME 20 minutes

FOR THE TART
150g/5½oz dark chocolate, 70% cocoa
 solids, broken into small pieces
4 eggs, lightly beaten
100g/3½oz/scant ½ cup caster/
 superfine sugar
75g/2½oz butter, melted
55g/2oz/scant ½ cup plain/all-purpose
 flour, sifted
23cm/9in shop-bought sweet pastry
 case

FOR THE SALTED CARAMEL SAUCE
100g/3½oz/heaped ½ cup soft light
 brown sugar
80g/2¾oz butter
55g/2oz golden/light corn syrup
125ml/4floz/½ cup double/heavy cream
1 tsp flaked sea salt, plus extra to taste

TO SERVE
icing/confectioners' sugar, for dusting
vanilla ice cream
dark and white chocolate

1 Preheat the oven to 180°C/350°F/gas 4.

2 To make the chocolate tart, put the chocolate in a large heatproof bowl. Rest the bowl over a pan of gently simmering water, so that the bottom of the bowl does not touch the water. Stir occasionally until the chocolate has melted. (Alternatively, melt the chocolate gently in the microwave.) Beat in the eggs, caster/superfine sugar, butter and flour.

3 Put the pastry case on a baking sheet, and pour in the chocolate filling. Bake for 15 minutes until just set. Leave to cool to room temperature. (The tart can be made a day ahead and left at room temperature, for a softer filling, or in the refrigerator for a firm-set tart.)

4 To make the sauce, melt the brown sugar, butter and golden/light corn syrup in a saucepan over a low heat. Bring to a simmer for about 3 minutes, swirling the pan a couple of times. Add the cream and salt and cook for a further minute. Taste (carefully, as it will be super hot) and add more salt, if you like. Transfer to a jug and leave to cool. (This can be made a few days ahead and kept in the refrigerator.)

5 When ready to serve, gently warm the sauce to a spoonable consistency and drizzle over slices of the tart. Using a vegetable peeler, slowly shave over lengths of the dark and white chocolate, creating little curls, then dust with icing/confectioners' sugar and add a scroll of ice cream sitting on the sugar to stop it from sliding around.

How to make
cheats' chocolate and salted caramel tart
If time really isn't on your side, there is nothing wrong with pimping up shop-bought products to create an impressive dessert. If you don't want to give the game away, just hide the packaging! Buy a simple **chocolate tart** or **torte** and cut into generous slices. Gently heat **1 tbsp shop-bought dulce de leche** or **caramel sauce** per person in the microwave to give you a spoonable consistency, then stir in **¼ tsp flaked sea salt** per person. Serve as above, and let your guests praise you for your creativity.

I love making brownies and adding exciting flavours to them. Chocolate and ginger is a wonderful combination and the stem ginger makes the finished result sticky, chewy and amazing! This makes a generous quantity so there's plenty for you to enjoy over a few days. Just store in an airtight container.

Chocolate and Ginger Brownies with Ginger Cream

MAKES 12 squares
PREPARATION TIME 20 minutes, plus cooling
COOKING TIME 25 minutes

FOR THE BROWNIES
200g/7oz butter, plus extra for greasing
200g/7oz dark chocolate, 70% cocoa solids, broken into small pieces
6 balls stem ginger, finely chopped
1 tsp sea salt
3 eggs
300g/10½oz/1⅓ cups granulated sugar
1 tsp vanilla extract
125g/4½oz/1 cup plain/all-purpose flour
1 tbsp unsweetened cocoa powder

FOR THE GINGER CREAM
200ml/7fl oz/scant 1 cup double/heavy or whipping cream
3 tbsp stem ginger syrup

1 Preheat the oven to 180°C/350°F/gas 4. Grease a deep 20x30cm/8x12in rectangular baking pan and line with baking paper.

2 Put the butter and chocolate in a large heatproof bowl. Rest the bowl over a pan of gently simmering water, so that the bottom of the bowl does not touch the water. Stir occasionally until the chocolate has melted. (Alternatively, melt the chocolate gently in the microwave.) Stir in the chopped ginger and salt.

3 Beat together the eggs, sugar and vanilla extract, using an electric mixer, until they are lovely and thick and creamy. Mix in the melted gingery chocolate. Finally sift in the flour and stir to combine. Pour into the prepared baking pan. Bake for 25 minutes until the top is cracking and the centre is just set. It may seem too soon to remove from the oven, but it will continue to cook when removed. As soon as you remove the pan from the oven, dust the top with the unsweetened cocoa powder.

4 Leave to cool in the pan for about 20 minutes before turning out and cutting into squares to save for later. (The brownies can be made a good few hours before you need them but keep them in a secret place so the kids can't get them.)

5 To make the cream, whisk together the cream and ginger syrup until it forms soft peaks.

6 Serve the brownies warm or cold with the ginger cream.

This is a stunning dessert and loses its impact if it's only small so I always make a large one. The guests appreciate it and we get lots left to enjoy the next day! As a treat for the kids, keep back some of the meringue and spoon small dollops (the size of a small walnut) onto a baking sheet. Put into the oven with the pavlova for just 1 hour. When cool, sandwich them together in pairs with a little whipped cream and jam or a chocolate spread to make what we call meringue kisses.

Limoncello and Blackberry Pavlova

MAKES 6–8 adult portions
PREPARATION TIME 20 minutes, plus
   cooling
COOKING TIME 1½ hours

4 egg whites
200g/7oz/scant 1 cup caster/
   superfine sugar
2 tsp cornflour/cornstarch
2 tsp lemon juice
250ml/9fl oz/1 cup double/heavy cream
4 tbsp limoncello liqueur
400g/14oz/2⅓ cups blackberries
grated lemon zest, to decorate

1 Preheat the oven to 140°C/275°F/gas 1 and line a baking sheet with non-stick baking paper.

2 Whisk the egg whites in a large bowl, using an electric mixer, until stiff peaks form. Mix together the sugar and cornflour/cornstarch, then whisk into the whites a spoonful at a time, adding the lemon juice with the last spoonful. Continue to whisk for a minute or so until the meringue is thick and glossy.

3 Spoon onto the prepared baking sheet and spread to form a circle about 22cm/8½in diameter, leaving a dip in the centre for the cream filling. Bake for about 1½ hours until the meringue is crisp. Leave to cool. (The meringue can be made 24 hours ahead of time and stored in an airtight container.)

4 To finish the pavlova, whisk the cream with the limoncello until it forms soft peaks. Reserve half of the blackberries for decoration, then lightly crush the rest with the back of a spoon. Fold into the cream and spoon into the centre of the pavlova. Top with the remaining berries, then sprinkle with grated lemon zest.

5 Serve within 1 hour of adding the cream.

How to make

chocolate pavlova
Simply add **25g/1oz/scant ¼ cup sifted unsweetened cocoa powder** with the sugar. For extra chocolatey loveliness, stir in **150g/5½oz milk chocolate drops** or **broken chocolate buttons**. Use plain whipped cream and mix in **raspberries**, **strawberries** or **canned cherries**. Decorate with **grated chocolate**.

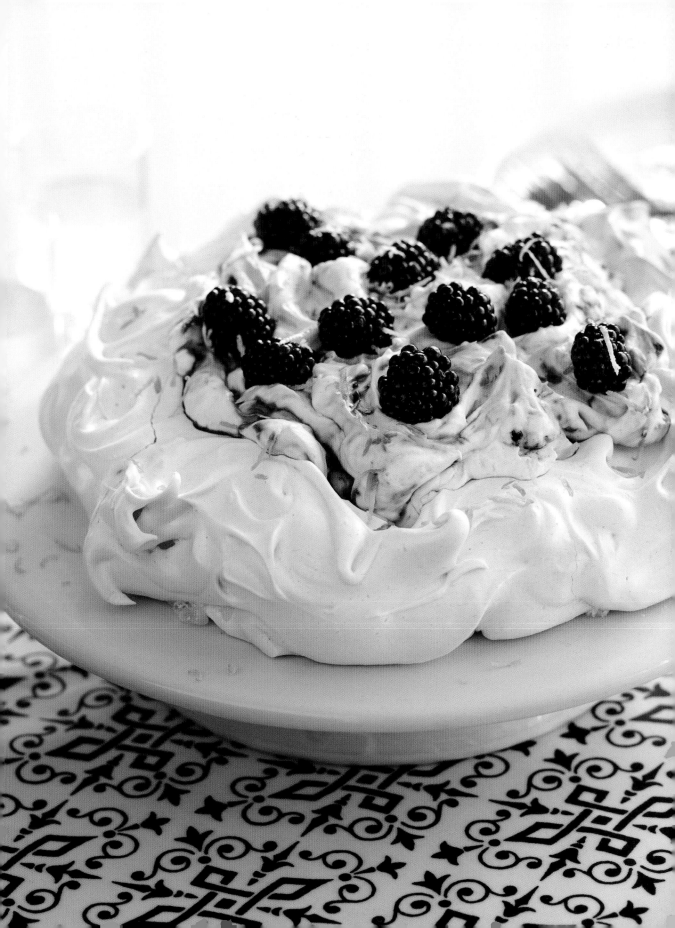

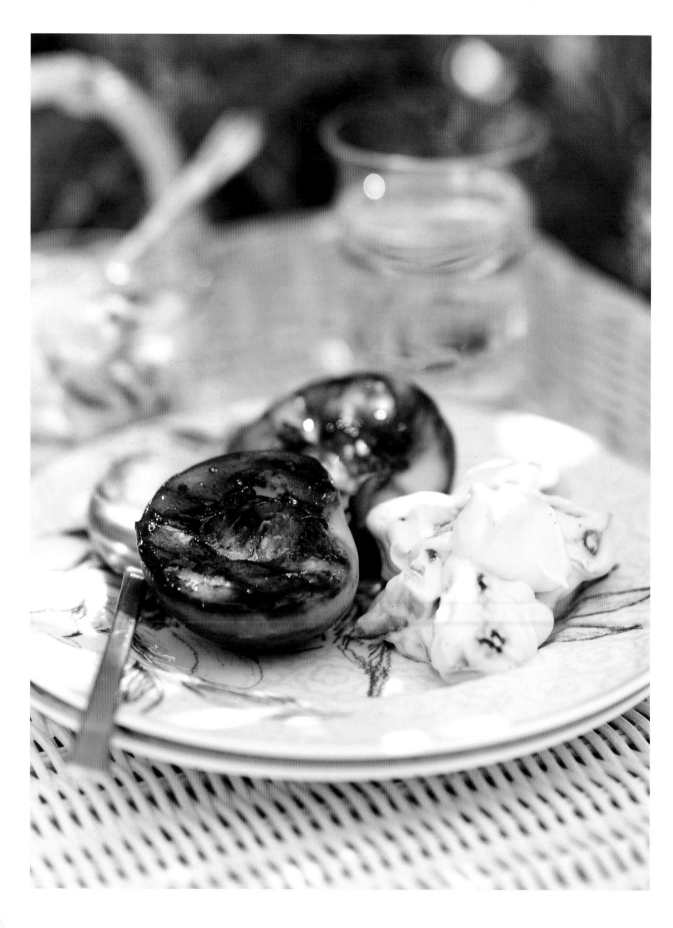

Cook these on the barbecue or use a griddle in the kitchen to make a light and refreshing end to a meal. Raspberries or a mixture of summer fruits can be used in place of the strawberries.

Griddled Peaches with Pimm's and Strawberry Cream

MAKES 4 adult portions
PREPARATION TIME 15 minutes, plus
  2 hours marinating
COOKING TIME 2 minutes

80ml/2½fl oz/⅓ cup Pimm's No.1 Cup
3 tbsp icing/confectioners' sugar, plus
  extra for dusting
1 vanilla pod/bean, halved and seeds
  removed
4 ripe peaches, halved and pitted
200ml/7fl oz/scant 1 cup double/heavy
  cream
200g/7oz/1⅓ cups strawberries, stalks
  removed and halved or quartered if
  large

1 Mix together the Pimm's, icing/confectioners' sugar and vanilla seeds. Put the peach halves in a shallow bowl, pour over the Pimm's mixture and cover with cling film/plastic wrap. Marinate the peaches in the refrigerator for a couple of hours or overnight if you can.

2 When you're ready to cook, put a griddle over a high heat or have your barbecue super hot. Lift the peaches out of the marinade and dust the cut sides with icing/confectioners' sugar. Put sugar-side down on the griddle or barbecue for 1 minute until the sugar has caramelized.

3 Put 3 tbsp of the marinade in a bowl and the rest in a small saucepan. Boil the syrup in the pan for 1 minute until it goes syrupy.

4 Meanwhile, whisk the cream with the reserved marinade until it just starts to form soft peaks.

5 Spoon the syrup over the peaches. Fold the strawberries through the cream and serve with the griddled peaches.

Leftovers for chocolate indulgence
vanilla hot chocolate
Most recipes tell you to put the leftover vanilla pod/bean in a jar of caster/superfine sugar to flavour it for baking. I like to keep one in a lidded container of fresh whole eggs. Keep them in the refrigerator and they will take on a subtle vanilla flavour through the porous shell, making them great for baking and sweet recipes.

I also like to treat myself to this indulgent hot chocolate when I get a moment to relax. To make 1 adult or 2 kid-sized cups, put **250ml/9fl oz/1 cup milk** in a saucepan with the **split and scraped vanilla pod/bean**. Very slowly bring to a simmer, stirring occasionally. The longer it takes, the more vanilla flavour will infuse into the milk. Remove from the heat and stir in **50g/1¾oz chopped dark chocolate, 70% cocoa solids**, until it has completely melted. Remove the vanilla pod/bean and pour the chocolate milk into your favourite cup. Serve as it is or, for an even bigger treat, top with **marshmallows** and **whipped cream**.

A light yet rich flourless cake that's ideal if you have to cater for someone who doesn't eat gluten, although you don't have to save it for them as the whole family will love it. It makes a large cake so there's plenty for leftovers to enjoy through the week.

Chocolate, Coconut and Raspberry Torte

MAKES 8 adult portions
PREPARATION TIME 15 minutes
COOKING TIME 40 minutes

175g/6oz butter, plus extra for greasing
175g/6oz dark chocolate, 70% cocoa solids, broken into small pieces
175g/6oz/heaped ¾ cup caster/superfine sugar
6 eggs, separated
175g/6oz/1¾ cups desiccated/dried shredded coconut, plus extra for sprinkling
150g/5½oz/1 cup raspberries
icing/confectioners' sugar, for dusting

1 Preheat the oven to 180°C/350°F/gas 4. Grease a 23cm/9in cake pan with butter and line the base with a circle of baking paper.

2 Put the chocolate in a large, heatproof bowl. Rest the bowl over a pan of gently simmering water, so that the bottom of the bowl does not touch the water. Stir occasionally until the chocolate has melted. (Alternatively, melt the chocolate gently in the microwave.)

3 Beat the butter and caster/superfine sugar, using an electric mixer, until light and creamy. Thoroughly beat in one egg yolk at a time, then add the melted chocolate and coconut, mixing until combined.

4 In a clean bowl, whisk the egg whites, using an electric mixer, until semi-stiff peaks form. Stir one-third into the chocolate mixture to soften the mixture, then gently fold in the remainder with a large metal spoon. Spoon into the prepared cake pan. Bake for 35–40 minutes until a skewer inserted into the centre comes out clean.

5 Leave to cool in the pan for 10 minutes, then transfer to a serving plate. Pile the raspberries on top and dust with icing/confectioners' sugar mixed with a little coconut.

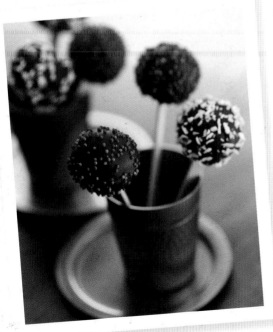

Leftovers for the kids
chocolate cake pops
If you have any torte left over, the kids will love you for ever if you make these. Break some of the **leftover torte** into fine crumbs and mix in just enough **raspberry jam** to bind together. Shape into truffle-sized balls and pop on a plate in the freezer for 15 minutes to chill. Dip the tip of lollipop sticks into a small bowl of **melted chocolate** (dark, milk or white) or **melted candy melts** and insert into the centre of the chilled balls. Then dip each cake pop into the melted chocolate/candy melts to cover evenly. Tap the stick to drip excess chocolate back into the bowl, then push the stick into something such as a piece of polystyrene or even a large potato with a flat base (this will bring back memories of cheese and pineapple on sticks). When the chocolate is almost but not quite set, scatter over some sprinkles and leave to set completely.

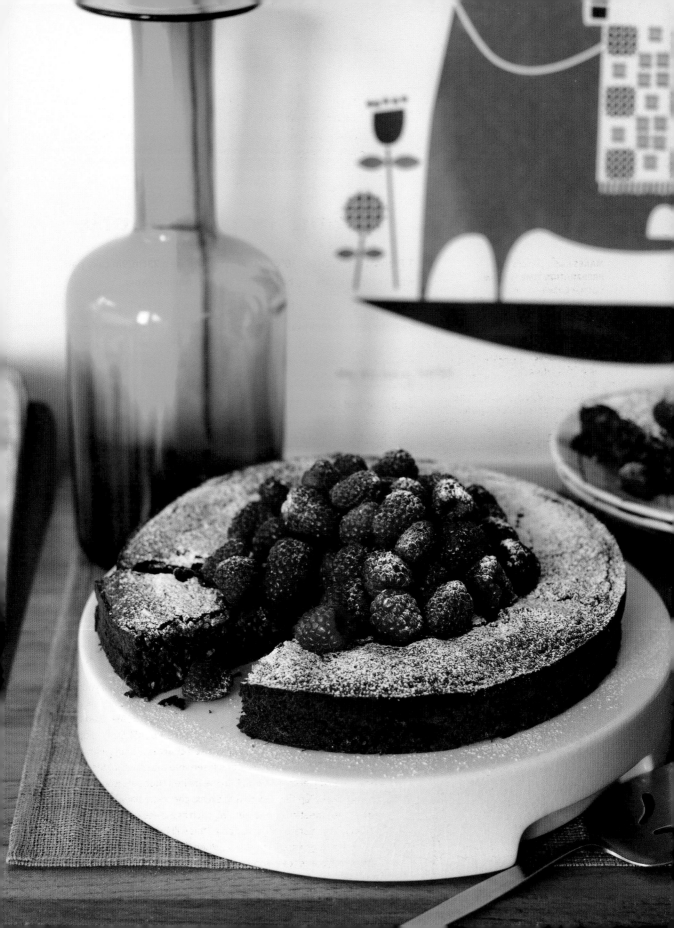

Index